Innovations in Fetal and Neonatal Surgery

Guest Editors

HANMIN LEE, MD
RONALD B. HIRSCHL, MD

CLINICS IN PERINATOLOGY

www.perinatology.theclinics.com

Consulting Editor

LUCKY JAIN, MD, MBA

June 2012 • Volume 39 • Number 2

SAUNDERS an imprint of ELSEVIER, Inc.

W.B. SAUNDERS COMPANY
A Division of Elsevier Inc.

Elsevier, Inc. • 1600 John F. Kennedy Blvd. • Suite 1800 • Philadelphia, PA 19103-2899

http://www.theclinics.com

CLINICS IN PERINATOLOGY Volume 39, Number 2
June 2012 ISSN 0095-5108, ISBN-13: 978-1-4557-3912-7

Editor: Kerry Holland
Developmental Editor: Donald Mumford

Clinics in Perinatology (ISSN 0095-5108) is published quarterly by Elsevier Inc., 360 Park Avenue South, New York, NY 10010-1710. Months of issue are March, June, September, and December. Business and Editorial Offices: 1600 John F. Kennedy Blvd., Ste. 1800, Philadelphia, PA 19103-2899. Customer Service Office: 3251 Riverport Lane, Maryland Heights, MO 63043. Periodicals postage paid at New York, NY and additional mailing offices. Subscription prices are $273.00 per year (US individuals), $401.00 per year (US institutions), $326.00 per year (Canadian individuals), $509.00 per year (Canadian institutions), $400.00 per year (foreign individuals), $509.00 per year (foreign institutions), $130.00 per year (US students), and $187.00 per year (Canadian and foreign students). Foreign air speed delivery is included in all Clinics subscription prices. All prices are subject to change without notice. **POSTMASTER:** Send address changes to *Clinics in Perinatology*, Elsevier Health Sciences Division, Subscription Customer Service, 3251 Riverport Lane, Maryland Heights, MO 63043. **Customer Service: Telephone: 1-800-654-2452** (U.S. and Canada); **1-314-447-8871** (outside U.S. and Canada). **Fax: 1-314-447-8029. E-mail: journalscustomerservice-usa@elsevier.com** (for print support); **journalsonlinesupport-usa@elsevier.com** (for online support).

Reprints. For copies of 100 or more, of articles in this publication, please contact the Commercial Reprints Department, Elsevier Inc., 360 Park Avenue South, New York, NY 10010-1710. Tel. (212) 633-3812; Fax: (212) 482-1935; E-mail: reprints@elsevier.com.

Clinics in Perinatology is also pubilshed in Spanish by McGraw-Hill Interamericana Editores S.A., P.O. Box 5-237, 06500 Mexico D.F., Mexico.

Clinics in Perinatology is covered in *MEDLINE/PubMed (Index Medicus) Current Contents, Excepta Medica, BIOSIS and ISI/BIOMED.*

Printed and bound by CPI Group (UK) Ltd, Croydon, CR0 4YY

Transferred to Digital Print 2012

Contributors

CONSULTING EDITOR

LUCKY JAIN, MD, MBA
Richard Blumberg Professor and Executive Vice Chairman, Department of Pediatrics, Emory University School of Medicine, Atlanta, Georgia

GUEST EDITORS

HANMIN LEE, MD
Professor of Clinical Surgery, Pediatrics, and Obstetrics, Gynecology & Reproductive Sciences, Chief, Division of Pediatric Surgery; Director, Fetal Treatment Center; Surgeon-in-Chief, UCSF Benioff Children's Hospital, San Francisco, California

RONALD B. HIRSCHL, MD
Arnold Coran Professor of Surgery, Head, Section of Pediatric Surgery, C.S. Mott Children's Hospital, Ann Arbor, Michigan

AUTHORS

KATHLEEN M. DOMINGUEZ, MD
Department of Surgery, Nationwide Children's Hospital, The Ohio State University College of Medicine, Columbus, Ohio

DIANA L. FARMER, MD, FAAP, FACS, FRCS
Pearl Stamps Stewart Professor and Chair, Division of Pediatric Surgery, Department of Surgery, School of Medicine; Surgeon-in-Chief, Children's Hospital, UC Davis Health System, University of California, Davis, Sacramento, California

ALAN W. FLAKE, MD
Professor of Surgery and Obstetrics and Gynecology, Department of Surgery, The Children's Center for Fetal Research, The Children's Hospital of Philadelphia, University of Pennsylvania School of Medicine, Philadelphia, Pennsylvania

JOHN E. FOKER, MD, PhD
Robert and Sharon Kaster Professor of Surgery, Division of Cardiovascular and Thoracic Surgery, University of Minnesota Medical School, Minneapolis, Minnesota; Scientific Director, Esophageal Atresia Treatment Program, Children's Hospital Boston, Harvard Medical School, Boston, Massachusetts

BRIAN W. GRAY, MD
Section of Pediatric Surgery, C.S. Mott Children's Hospital, University of Michigan Health System, Ann Arbor, Michigan

MICHAEL HARRISON, MD
Division of Pediatric Surgery, Department of Surgery, Fetal Treatment Center, University of California, San Francisco, San Francisco, California

RICHARD S. HERMAN, MD
Clinical Lecturer, Section of Critical Care, Division of Pediatric Surgery, University of Michigan, Ann Arbor, Michigan

SHINJIRO HIROSE, MD
Assistant Professor of Surgery, Division of Pediatric Surgery, Department of Surgery, Fetal Treatment Center, University of California, San Francisco, San Francisco, California

SALEEM ISLAM, MD, MPH
Associate Professor of Surgery and Pediatrics, Pediatric Surgery, Department of Surgery, University of Florida College of Medicine, Gainesville, Florida

SHAUN M. KUNISAKI, MD, MSc
Assistant Professor, Department of Surgery, Fetal Diagnosis and Treatment Center, C.S. Mott Children's Hospital and Von Voigtlander Women's Hospital, University of Michigan Medical School, Ann Arbor, Michigan

JEAN-MARTIN LABERGE, MD, FRCSC, FACS
Professor of Surgery, Pediatric Surgery, Montreal Children's Hospital, McGill University Health Center, Montreal, Quebec, Canada

KEVIN P. LALLY, MD, MS
A.G. McNeese Chair in Pediatric Surgery, Richard Andrassy Distinguished Professor, Chairman, Department of Pediatric Surgery, The University of Texas, School of Medicine at Houston; Surgeon-in-Chief, Children's Memorial Hermann Hospital, Houston, Texas

HANMIN LEE, MD
Professor of Clinical Surgery, Pediatrics, and Obstetrics, Gynecology & Reproductive Sciences, Chief, Division of Pediatric Surgery; Director, Fetal Treatment Center; Surgeon-in-Chief, UCSF Benioff Children's Hospital, San Francisco, California

TIPPI C. MACKENZIE, MD
Assistant Professor of Surgery, Eli and Edythe Broad Center of Regeneration Medicine and Stem Cell Research, Department of Surgery, San Francisco, California

DOUG MINIATI, MD
Assistant Professor, Division of Pediatric Surgery, Department of Surgery, Fetal Treatment Center, University of California, San Francisco, San Francisco, California

R. LAWRENCE MOSS, MD
Department of Surgery, Nationwide Children's Hospital, The Ohio State University College of Medicine, Columbus, Ohio

GEORGE B. MYCHALISKA, MD
Section of Pediatric Surgery, Fetal Diagnosis and Treatment Center, C.S. Mott Children's Hospital, University of Michigan Health System, Ann Arbor, Michigan

AMAR NIJAGAL, MD
Postdoctoral Research Fellow, Eli and Edythe Broad Center of Regeneration Medicine and Stem Cell Research, Department of Surgery, San Francisco, California

PRAMOD S. PULIGANDLA, MD, MSc, FRCSC, FACS, FAAP
Associate Professor of Surgery and Pediatrics, Program Director, Pediatric Surgery, Montreal Children's Hospital, McGill University Health Center, McGill University, Montreal, Quebec, Canada

PAYAM SAADAI, MD
Division of Pediatric Surgery, Department of Surgery, Fetal Treatment Center, University of California, San Francisco, San Francisco, California

ANDREW W. SHAFFER, MD, MS
Section of Pediatric Surgery, C.S. Mott Children's Hospital, University of Michigan Health System, Ann Arbor; Department of Surgery, William Beaumont Health System, Detroit, Michigan

EVELINE H. SHUE, MD
Resident, Division of Pediatric Surgery, Department of Surgery, Fetal Treatment Center, University of California, San Francisco, San Francisco, California

DANIEL H. TEITELBAUM, MD
Professor of Surgery, Section of Pediatric Surgery, University of Michigan, Ann Arbor, Michigan

KUOJEN TSAO, MD
Assistant Professor, Departments of Pediatric Surgery and Surgery, The University of Texas School of Medicine at Houston; The Children's Memorial Hermann Hospital, Houston, Texas

Contents

This article reviews fetal intervention for congenital anomalies, which has evolved from a mere concept to a medical specialty over the past 3 decades. Advances in surgical techniques have paralleled developments in fetal imaging, fetal diagnosis, and the advent of maternal tocolysis to prevent preterm labor. Fetal intervention has become an important option for fetuses who would otherwise not survive gestation or who would endure significant morbidity and mortality after birth. However, there were many trials and tribulations as fetal surgery developed into a medical specialty.

Myelomeningocele (MMC) is a congenital neural tube defect that occurs in approximately 1 in 2900 live births in the United States. It is a devastating disability with significant morbidity and mortality within the first few decades of life. MMC was the first nonlethal disease to be considered and studied for fetal surgery and is now the most common open fetal surgery performed. The recently completed MOMS randomized controlled trial has shown that fetal repair for MMC can improve hydrocephalus and hindbrain herniation, can reduce the need for vetriculoperitoneal shunting, and may improve distal neurologic function in some patients.

Congenital diaphragmatic hernia (CDH) is a common birth anomaly. Absence or presence of liver herniation and determination of lung-to-head ratio are the most accurate predictors of prognosis for fetuses with CDH. Though open fetal CDH repair has been abandoned, fetal endoscopic balloon tracheal occlusion promotes lung growth in fetuses with severe CDH. Although significant improvements in lung function have not yet been shown in humans, reversible or dynamic tracheal occlusion is promising for select fetuses with severe CDH. This article reviews advances in prenatal diagnosis of CDH, the experimental basis for tracheal occlusion, and its translation into human clinical trials.

In utero hematopoietic cell transplantation (IUHCTx) is a promising strategy for the treatment of common hematopoietic disorders and for inducing immune tolerance in the fetus. Although the efficacy of IUHCTx has been demonstrated in multiple small and large animal models, the clinical application of this technique in humans has had limited success. Recent studies in mice have demonstrated that the maternal immune system plays a critical role in limiting engraftment in the fetus. This article reviews the therapeutic rationale of IUHCTx, potential barriers to its applications, and recent experimental strategies to improve its clinical success.

This review addresses the history and evolution of neonatal extracorporeal membrane oxygenation (ECMO), with a discussion of the indications, contraindications, modalities, outcomes, and impact of ECMO. Controversies surrounding novel uses of ECMO in neonates, namely ECMO for premature infants and ex utero intrapartum therapy with transition to ECMO, are discussed. The development of an extracorporeal artificial placenta for support of premature infants is presented, including the rationale, research, and challenges. ECMO has had a dramatic effect on the care of critically ill neonates over the past 4 decades, and there is great potential to expand these benefits in the future.

Confusion, controversy, and uncertainty are all terms applicable to the diagnosis and management of congenital lung lesions both prenatally and postnatally. This review examines the current status of fetal diagnosis and treatment of these lesions; reviews the various classifications, including congenital cystic adenomatoid malformation/congenital pulmonary airway malformation, sequestrations, variants and hybrid lesions; discusses the risk of malignant transformation or misdiagnosis with pleuropulmonary blastoma; presents the arguments in favor and against resection of asymptomatic lesions, the timing of such resection, and the long-term pulmonary function after resection; and reviews the experience with thoracoscopic resection of congenital lung lesions.

This article focuses on selected topics in the diagnosis and management of patients with esophageal atresia (EA) with or without tracheoesophageal fistula. The current status of prenatal diagnosis and recent advances in surgical techniques, including thoracoscopic repair for short-gap EA and tension-induced esophageal growth for long-gap EA, are reviewed.

Although no consensus exists among pediatric surgeons regarding the role of these procedures in the treatment of EA, one can reasonably expect that, as they evolve, their application will become more widespread in this challenging patient population.

GOAL STATEMENT

The goal of *Clinics in Perinatology* is to keep practicing neonatologists and maternal-fetal medicine specialists up to date with current clinical practice in perinatology by providing timely articles reviewing the state of the art in patient care.

ACCREDITATION

The *Clinics in Perinatology* is planned and implemented in accordance with the Essential Areas and Policies of the Accreditation Council for Continuing Medical Education (ACCME) through the joint sponsorship of the University of Virginia School of Medicine and Elsevier. The University of Virginia School of Medicine is accredited by the ACCME to provide continuing medical education for physicians.

The University of Virginia School of Medicine designates this enduring material activity for a maximum of 15 *AMA PRA Category 1 Credit*(s)™ for each issue, 60 credits per year. Physicians should only claim credit commensurate with the extent of their participation in the activity.

The American Medical Association has determined that physicians not licensed in the US who participate in this CME enduring material activity *are eligible* for a maximum of 15 *AMA PRA Category 1 Credit*(s)™ for each issue, 60 credits per year.

Credit can be earned by reading the text material, taking the CME examination online at http://www.theclinics.com/home/cme, and completing the evaluation. After taking the test, you will be required to review any and all incorrect answers. Following completion of the test and evaluation, your credit will be awarded and you may print your certificate.

FACULTY DISCLOSURE/CONFLICT OF INTEREST

The University of Virginia School of Medicine, as an ACCME accredited provider, endorses and strives to comply with the Accreditation Council for Continuing Medical Education (ACCME) Standards of Commercial Support, Commonwealth of Virginia statutes, University of Virginia policies and procedures, and associated federal and private regulations and guidelines on the need for disclosure and monitoring of proprietary and financial interests that may affect the scientific integrity and balance of content delivered in continuing medical education activities under our auspices.

The University of Virginia School of Medicine requires that all CME activities accredited through this institution be developed independently and be scientifically rigorous, balanced and objective in the presentation/discussion of its content, theories and practices.

All authors/editors participating in an accredited CME activity are expected to disclose to the readers relevant financial relationships with commercial entities occurring within the past 12 months (such as grants or research support, employee, consultant, stock holder, member of speakers bureau, etc.). The University of Virginia School of Medicine will employ appropriate mechanisms to resolve potential conflicts of interest to maintain the standards of fair and balanced education to the reader. Questions about specific strategies can be directed to the Office of Continuing Medical Education, University of Virginia School of Medicine, Charlottesville, Virginia.

The faculty and staff of the University of Virginia Office of Continuing Medical Education have no financial affiliations to disclose.

The authors/editors listed below have identified no professional or financial affiliations for themselves or their spouse/partner:

Robert Boyle, MD (Test Author); Kathleen M. Dominguez, MD; Diana L. Farmer, MD, FAAP, FACS, FRCS; Alan W. Flake, MD; John E. Foker, MD, PhD; Brian W. Gray, MD; Michael Harrison, MD; Richard S. Herman, MD; Shinjiro Hirose, MD; Ronald B. Hirschl, MD (Guest Editor); Kerry Holland, (Acquisitions Editor); Saleem Islam, MD, MPH; Lucky Jain, MD, MBA (Consulting Editor); Shaun M. Kunisaki, MD, MSc; Jean-Martin Laberge, MD, FRCSC, FACS; Kevin P. Lally, MD, MS; Hanmin Lee, MD (Guest Editor); Tippi C. MacKenzie, MD; Doug Miniati, MD; R. Lawrence Moss, MD; George B. Mychaliska, MD; Amar Nijagal, MD; Pramod S. Puligandla, MD, MSc, FRCSC, FACS, FAAP; Payam Saadai, MD; Andrew W. Shaffer, MD, MS; Eveline H. Shue, MD; Daniel H. Teitelbaum, MD; and KuoJen Tsao, MD.

Disclosure of Discussion of Non-FDA Approved Uses for Pharmaceutical Products and/or Medical Devices

The University of Virginia School of Medicine, as an ACCME provider, requires that all faculty presenters identify and disclose any off-label uses for pharmaceutical and medical device products. The University of Virginia School of Medicine recommends that each physician fully review all the available data on new products or procedures prior to clinical use.

TO ENROLL

To enroll in the Clinics in Perinatology Continuing Medical Education program, call customer service at 1-800-654-2452 or visit us online at www.theclinics.com/home/cme. The CME program is available to subscribers for an additional fee of $196.00

CLINICS IN PERINATOLOGY

Foreword

The Surgical Neonate: We Need to Track Outcomes

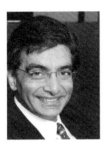

Lucky Jain, MD, MBA
Consulting Editor

It is hard to argue with the tremendous gains that have been made in improving care of newborns undergoing surgical procedures. Prenatal ultrasounds and other advanced diagnostic approaches have allowed for more accurate timing and scope of surgical interventions.[1] Minimally invasive surgical procedures have become more popular.[2] Anesthesia and pain control have become more precise, as have postoperative support and infection control. Neonatologists and surgeons work in teams, much more than they did a decade or two ago. These and many other improvements have led to a steady reduction in intraoperative and postoperative complications. However, questions linger about many aspects of the care and outcomes. Is fetal surgery beneficial, are general anesthetics too toxic to the growing brain, should we do a laparotomy or put in a drain, should we ligate that pesky ductus or let Mother Nature take its course? The list goes on.[3,4]

Whether or not to call the surgeon is a decision that often falls into the lap of the neonatologist, who is also tasked with safeguarding the overall intact survival of a vulnerable newborn. For many conditions where surgery used to be the standard of care, new doubts have surfaced. For example, after decades of chasing the patent ductus arteriosus with medical and surgical approaches, new evidence suggests that it might be safer to leave the ductus alone.[5,6] While physiologic parameters may improve after ligation of a symptomatic ductus, the impact on the long-term outcome is less clear. Is it because the cumulative surgical risks and complications, and the cardiac effects of sudden changes in afterload, overwhelm any potential gain from eliminating the left to right shunt?[6] How do we identify infants for whom the benefits of ligation will outweigh these risks? Do we need a randomized controlled trial to answer this question? If so, will there be enough equipoise to provide for meaningful randomization of all eligible patients?

Clin Perinatol 39 (2012) xiii–xiv
doi:10.1016/j.clp.2012.05.002
0095-5108/12/$ – see front matter © 2012 Elsevier Inc. All rights reserved.

And then the vexing issue of intestinal perforation: a lap or a drain?[3] With little more than shaky evidence supporting either of these two approaches as superior, clinicians have stuck to their own preferences. A recent analysis of the published literature concluded that there were not any significant advantages or harms in inserting a drain over surgically opening the abdomen; however, there is too little evidence to fully understand the risks and benefits of this approach.[3] More evidence is needed, but clinical trials have had a hard time enrolling patients, and we are far from an evidence-based answer. Meanwhile, the incidence of spontaneous intestinal perforation and perforation associated with necrotizing enterocolitis shows no signs of decreasing.

This issue of the *Clinics in Perinatology* represents an impressive lineup of reviews addressing these and many other common surgical issues in the neonatal period. I want to thank the editors and authors for a superb collection of articles and Kerry Holland at Elsevier for supporting their publication. The singular message one sees emerging is the need to focus on outcomes; it is only with rigorous tracking and sharing of outcomes data that we will be able to identify best practices that promote intact survival of our most vulnerable surgical patients.

Lucky Jain, MD, MBA
Department of Pediatrics
Emory University School of Medicine
2015 Uppergate Drive
Atlanta, GA 30322, USA

E-mail address:
ljain@emory.edu

REFERENCES

1. Collins SL, Impey L. Prenatal diagnosis: types and techniques. Early Hum Dev 2012;88:3–8.
2. Kuebler JF, Ure BM. Minimally invasive surgery in the neonate. Semin Fetal Neonatal Med 2011;16:151–6.
3. Rao SC, Basani L, Simmer K, et al. Peritoneal drain versus laparotomy as initial surgical treatment for perforated nectrotizing enterocolitis or spontaneous intestinal perforation in preterm low birth weight infants. Cochrane Database Syst Rev 2011;15:CD006182.
4. Noori S. Pros and cons of patent ductus arteriosus ligation: hemodynamic changes and other morbidities after patent ductus arteriosus ligation. Semin Perinatol 2012;36:139–45.
5. McNamara PJ, Stewart L, Shivananda SP, et al. Patent ductus arteriosus ligation is associated with impaired left ventricular systolic performance in premature infants weighing less than 1000 g. J Thorac Cardiovasc Surg 2010;140:150–7.
6. Clyman RI, Couto J, Murphy GM. Patent ductus arteriosus: are current neonatal treatment options better or worse than no treatment at all. Semin Perinatol 2012; 36:123–9.

Preface

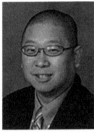 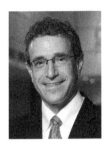

Hanmin Lee, MD   Ronald B. Hirschl, MD
Guest Editors

We are pleased in this edition of *Clinics in Perinatology* to present advances in fetal and neonatal surgery from internationally renowned leaders. The core aspect of the field of pediatric surgery is the care of neonates with acquired and congenital anomalies that may require surgical intervention. With the development of specialized neonatal intensive care units, pediatric surgeons developed surgical techniques and were able to achieve anatomic repair of even the most complex of neonatal anomalies. Many anomalies were effectively treated by early leaders in pediatric surgery with postnatal surgical correction of the anatomic defect. For example, most infants with intestinal atresia require one surgery and have essentially normal lifelong function. However, for other diseases, outcomes are often adversely affected by infant comorbidities, lack of adequate replacement tissue, and progressive physiologic perturbations from the anatomic anomalies. For example, while the anatomic defect in congenital diaphragmatic hernia can be repaired effectively postnatally, pulmonary hypoplasia and pulmonary hypotension cause significant morbidity and mortality. This issue focuses on recent prenatal and postnatal surgical advances for complex diseases managed by perinatologists, neonatologists, and pediatric surgeons to improve not only survival but also long-term outcomes.

Advances in fetal diagnosis have allowed clinicians to accurately identify most complex anomalies prenatally, and increasingly, stratify the severity of many diseases. In many instances, diagnoses are made in the second trimester and clinicians can give affected families significantly improved outcomes data. Informed families are able to make more informed decisions about the pregnancy and delivery plans. In some cases, fetal intervention may ameliorate some of the progressive physiologic organ damage that occurs from congenital anomalies. Drs Shue, Harrison, and Hirose discuss general aspects of fetal diagnosis and therapy. The field of fetal surgery has progressed from small case series to international multicenter registries and multicenter, prospective randomized controlled trials. Drs Saadai and Farmer discuss diagnosis and treatment of fetal myelomengincole, including the outcomes from the MOMS trial, which was recently awarded the prestigious Trial of the Year by the Society for Clinical Trials and Project ImpACT. Drs Shue, Miniati, and Lee discuss fetal diagnosis and therapy for congenital diaphragmatic hernia, including ongoing work on fetoscopic tracheal occlusion to promote fetal lung growth. Drs Nijagal, Flake, and Mackenzie present work from their laboratories and others on the current state

Clin Perinatol 39 (2012) xv–xvi
doi:10.1016/j.clp.2012.05.001   **perinatology.theclinics.com**

of fetal stem cell transplantation. This is a particularly exciting field that may leverage the relatively underdeveloped state of the fetal immune system.

Drs Puligandla and Laberge bridge prenatal and postnatal diagnosis and therapy with their article on advances in the treatment of congenital lung lesions. Classification, diagnosis, and treatment of lung lesions have undergone significant advances over the last decade.

Drs Gray, Shaffer, and Mychaliska blur the lines between prenatal and postnatal physiology with their groundbreaking work on advances in ECMO and artificial placenta. Significant advances continue in the postnatal diagnosis and treatment of complex neonatal anomalies. Dr Moss, who led the landmark prospective randomized controlled trial comparing perintoneal drainage to laporotomy for severe necrotizing enterocolitis, discusses further advances in the treatment of NEC along with colleague Dr Dominguez. Drs Herman and Teitelbaum discuss advances in the management of anorectal anomalies, while Drs Kunisaki and Foker discuss advances in the treatment of esophageal atresia, including their highly innovative work on esophageal lengthening for esophageal atresia allowing for primary repairs. Drs Tsao and Lally highlight postnatal advances in the care of infants with CDH, including critical lessons learned from leading the international CDH registry, and Dr Islam reviews advances in the field of abdominal wall defects, including both gastroschisis and omphalocele.

The field of pediatric surgery has been a wonderful incubator for innovations in medicine that start from clinical needs for patient care and then through the hard work of many become clinical reality. Examples of significant innovations include the establishment of angiogenesis as a critical component of nearly every aspect of medically related basic science research led by Dr Judah Folkman. Dr Robert Bartlett's work on ECMO is currently continued by the holder of the Bartlett chair and one of this edition's authors, George Mychaliska. Dr Joseph "Jay" Vacanti helped found the field of tissue engineering, which increasingly is finding clinical applications throughout medicine. Dr Lucian Leape was an innovator in improving processes for safety in medicine, which has broad application throughout all aspects of medicine. Dr Michael Harrison is widely considered the father of fetal surgery and currently is a leader in pediatric device acceleration. These are just a few examples of innovation by pediatric surgeons that have successfully translated to improved patient care for patients of all ages, but generally started with a focused need for neonates. The care of neonatal surgical diseases continues to be a source of significant innovation in medicine. This edition outlines some of the recent advances in fetal and neonatal surgery as presented by international leaders.

Hanmin Lee, MD
Division of Pediatric Surgery
Fetal Treatment Center, UCSF Benioff Children's Hospital
513 Parnassus Avenue, HSW 1601
San Francisco, CA 94143, USA

Ronald B. Hirschl, MD
Section of Pediatric Surgery
C.S. Mott Children's Hospital
1500 East Medical Center Drive
F3970 Mott Children's Hospital
Ann Arbor, MI 48109-0245, USA

E-mail addresses:
leeh@surgery.ucsf.edu (H. Lee)
rhirschl@med.umich.edu (R.B. Hirschl)

Maternal-Fetal Surgery
History and General Considerations

Eveline H. Shue, MD, Michael Harrison, MD, Shinjiro Hirose, MD*

KEYWORDS

- History of fetal surgery • History of prenatal intervention
- Considerations for fetal treatment programs

KEY POINTS

- Fetal intervention was made possible by advances in technology that allowed accurate diagnosis, and reliable monitoring of mother and fetus. Further advances in minimally invasive surgery and miniaturization of instruments have allowed interventions to move away from open surgery to percutaneous procedures.
- Techniques for fetal intervention were tested in vivo in various animal models in order to perform "proof of concept" testing. Further experimentation led to interventions that treat physiological abnormalities, not just anatomic ones.
- A multi-disciplinary team is critical for successful fetal intervention. From beginning to end, starting with patient counseling, to performance of any procedure, to post-operative monitoring and follow up, the integration of multiple specialties is necessary.
- New fetal treatment programs should be initiated with adequate oversight and resources to ensure success and safety for both mother and unborn child.

INTRODUCTION

Fetal intervention for congenital anomalies has evolved from a mere concept to a medical specialty over the past 3 decades. Techniques used in fetal surgery, such as open hysterotomy, fetal endoscopy, and image-guided percutaneous procedures, were first developed in animal models before application in human patients. Advances in surgical techniques paralleled developments in fetal imaging, fetal diagnosis, and the advent of maternal tocolysis to prevent preterm labor. Fetal intervention has become an important option for fetuses who would otherwise not survive gestation or who would endure significant morbidity and mortality after birth. However, there were many trials and tribulations as fetal surgery developed into a medical specialty. This article reviews its history as well as general considerations in establishing a fetal treatment program.

Division of Pediatric Surgery, Department of Surgery, Fetal Treatment Center, University of California, San Francisco, 513 Parnassus Avenue, HSW-1601, San Francisco, CA 94143-0570, USA
* Corresponding author.
E-mail address: shinjiro.hirose@ucsfmedctr.org

Clin Perinatol 39 (2012) 269–278
doi:10.1016/j.clp.2012.04.010
0095-5108/12/$ – see front matter Published by Elsevier Inc.

LAYING THE FOUNDATION

Fetal development was first observed in animals and described in the late 1800s. However, animal models simulating human congenital anomalies, such as diaphragmatic hernia in the fetal lamb[1] and hydronephrosis in the rabbit[2] and lamb,[3] were not developed until the 1960s and 1970s. These models allowed scientists to study normal fetal development and physiology as well as the pathophysiology behind these anomalies. Congenital diaphragmatic hernia (CDH) and congenital hydronephrosis are both examples of simple anatomic malformations that interfere with normal organ development. If these anatomic malformations could be corrected antenatally, fetal lung and kidney development could potentially proceed normally.

Early attempts at fetal intervention in humans transpired even before prenatal monitoring and diagnostic techniques had been developed. Sir William Liley described the first human fetal intervention in the 1960s in New Zealand. He demonstrated that in utero intra-abdominal transfusion of blood in the fetus could treat severe hemolytic anemia from immune-mediated hydrops.[4] Around the same time, obstetricians in New York and Puerto Rico tried to access fetal circulation for complete exchange transfusion to treat hydrops fetalis.[5,6] These investigators exposed the fetus through a hysterotomy and cannulated the femoral and jugular vessels. However, their experience was discouraging and open fetal surgery was abandoned for the next decade. These initial experiences introduced the concept of fetal intervention,[7] but progress in the field had to wait until better anesthetic agents, imaging modalities, animal models, and surgical techniques had been developed.

ENABLING FACTORS

The ability to monitor the fetus throughout gestation and during a potential fetal intervention was crucial to the development of fetal surgery as a medical specialty. The first crude measurements of fetal well-being were subjective reports of fetal movement from the mother or palpation by the obstetrician. Subsequently the fetal heart beat, detected first by auscultation and then by electric monitors, was used to assess fetal well-being and distress. Gestational hormones detected in the maternal blood and urine correlated with the condition of the fetus, whereas chromosome abnormalities, inherited metabolic disorders, and fetal lung maturity could be diagnosed through amniocentesis (analysis of fetal cells in the amniotic fluid). Development of these diagnostic tools allowed physicians to monitor fetal well-being and diagnose anomalies before birth.

Development of a safe, noninvasive imaging technique for the diagnosis of fetal anomalies was especially crucial for the evolution of fetal intervention. Radiation from x-rays was potentially harmful to the developing fetus, and injection of radiopaque material into the amniotic fluid for an amniogram was an invasive technique, which did not accurately delineate fetal anatomy and which furthermore increased the risk of premature rupture of membranes and preterm labor. Ultrasonography, however, was safe, noninvasive, and accurately defined normal and abnormal fetal anatomy with considerable detail. Using prenatal ultrasonography, sonographers were able to visualize the developing heart and valves, assess fetal growth, and identify anatomic abnormalities. Ultrasonography could also be used to guide diagnostic procedures, such as amniocentesis and, later, more invasive procedures such as fetal shunt placement or fetal percutaneous umbilical cord blood sampling. The advent of ultrasonography in the late 1950s and early 1960s gave physicians a window into the uterus to examine the developing fetus, and enabled them to define the natural history of normal gestation and congenital anomalies without harming the mother or fetus.

The natural history and pathophysiology behind many congenital anomalies, such as hydronephrosis, diaphragmatic hernia, and hydrops fetalis, was defined using serial sonographic studies. These observations initiated discussions about whether fetal interventions could alter the natural course of fetal development in patients with these anomalies. Pediatric surgeons, obstetricians, obstetric sonologists, perinatologists, and neonatologists interested in managing the mother and fetus throughout pregnancy and improving postnatal outcomes began to theorize about the optimal timing for potential prenatal treatments and the mode of delivery for fetuses with anomalies. These collaborative interactions were the foundation for the study and practice of fetal medicine. Before these ideas could be tried in humans, however, the physiologic rationale and feasibility of in utero repair needed to be established in animal models.[8,9]

ANIMAL MODELS

Advances in the ability to detect fetal anomalies through ultrasound in conjunction with the advent of animal models launched the field of fetal medicine. The fetal lamb model of CDH is perhaps the best model that parallels the evolution of fetal surgery. Surgical creation of a diaphragmatic defect in fetal lambs replicated the phenotype seen in human infants with CDH: a diaphragmatic hernia, pulmonary hypoplasia, and pulmonary hypertension.[4,10] This model has been used over the past 3 decades to study the natural history of CDH and to develop fetal interventions to treat pulmonary hypoplasia caused by congenital diaphragmatic hernia. In utero repair of diaphragmatic hernia,[10] open fetal tracheal occlusion,[11] and subsequently, fetal endoscopic balloon tracheal occlusion[12] were all successfully developed in the fetal lamb model of CDH before translation into fetal intervention in humans.

In 1978, investigators at the University of California, San Francisco (UCSF) began to perform experiments directed toward fetal therapy. Significant enthusiasm led to exploration of new therapies for obstructive uropathy, CDH, and hydrocephalus. Initially experiments were conducted in fetal lamb models of CDH and urinary tract obstruction. The pathophysiology of these anomalies was reproduced with simple, surgically created anatomic defects in the animals, and the physiologic and developmental sequelae were documented before and after surgical repair. This pattern of investigation continued over the next 2 decades, and established the fetal lamb model as the most widely used and accepted method of testing the physiologic rationale for fetal intervention in several congenital anomalies.

The fetal lamb model of gestation is ideal for experimental investigation because the sheep uterus is resistant to uterine contractions and labor in response to surgical manipulation. By the same token, however, this model was incomplete for developing human in utero intervention because the human uterus is sensitive to preterm labor. Safety for both the mother and the fetus had to be established in a nonhuman primate model before translation into human therapy. UCSF was the first to conduct fetal surgery experiments in rhesus monkeys, followed by the Primate Colony at the University of California, Davis. At UC Davis, primates that underwent fetal surgery were studied for years afterward to determine the effects of fetal intervention on future fertility and reproductive potential. Access to facilities that were equipped for experiments in fetal lambs and primates was crucial to the development of techniques for fetal intervention and fetal surgery as a medical specialty.

THE EARLY DAYS: UCSF AND BEYOND

Congenital hydronephrosis was the first fetal anomaly to be considered for human fetal intervention. It was easily detected using ultrasonography, and the pathophysiology was well defined. Without intervention, obstruction of the posterior urethral valves caused urinary retention in the bladder. Not only did this cause hydronephrosis and impair normal renal development but also led to oligohydramnios and pulmonary hypoplasia, causing respiratory distress in the neonate at birth. These physiologic sequelae had been documented in humans and subsequently demonstrated in laboratory experiments to be reversible by simple fetal bladder decompression before birth. Using a double-pigtail shunt for percutaneous fetal bladder decompression developed by pediatric surgeon Michael Harrison, a multidisciplinary UCSF team comprising Harrison, perinatologist Mickey Golbus, and sonologist Roy Filly became the first to treat congenital hydronephrosis due to posterior urethral valves.[13] The technique, device, and patient-selection criteria have all evolved over time, but this initial successful operation was a landmark in fetal surgery, a feasible and effective procedure that was safe for both the mother and the fetus.

Between 1982 and 1983 in Denver, a ventriculoamniotic shunt was placed for obstructive hydrocephalus,[14] and a vesicoamniotic shunt and open fetal surgery was performed for obstructive uropathy at UCSF. A growing number of procedures were being performed at several other centers in the United States, and the pioneers of fetal surgery recognized that they would have to proceed cautiously. Unwanted publicity would raise ethical issues and significantly skew public perception. Around the world, physicians dedicated to fetal medicine agreed that ethical standards and guidelines for fetal intervention needed to be established.

In 1982, The Kroc Foundation hosted a conference called "Unborn: Management of the Fetus with a Correctable Defect" to discuss ethical guidelines and standards for treatment. Perinatal obstetricians, surgeons, ultrasonologists, pediatricians, bioethicists, and physiologists from 13 centers across 5 countries convened to review experimental evidence and clinical experience with fetal intervention.[15] The participants discussed the potential risks and benefits of fetal intervention, problems to avoid, and future directions for the field. This collaborative scientific community also agreed to share experience and information, start a registry of fetal cases, and formulate guidelines for patient selection and treatment. This meeting was the foundation for the International Fetal Medicine and Surgery Society (IFMSS), which began publishing a professional journal, Fetal Diagnosis & Therapy, and hosting annual meetings to exchange and share information.

The framework set by the IFMSS was one of excellence, scientific inquiry, and integrity. This community was dedicated to publishing both good and poor outcomes as a result of fetal intervention. The registry of fetal cases resulted in a publication of early results of fetal catheter shunts for hydrocephalus and obstructive uropathy in the New England Journal of Medicine.[16] While outcomes of fetal catheter shunts for obstructive uropathy were encouraging, outcomes from catheter shunts for hydrocephalus were less positive, with a procedure-related mortality of 10%. Given these discouraging results, fetal surgeons and the IFMSS community voluntarily moved away from catheter shunts for fetal hydrocephalus. To this day, IFMSS continues to be a collaborative community that consistently reevaluates experience with fetal surgery using the highest scientific standards.

FETAL SURGERY MATURES: TRIALS AND TRIBULATIONS

The fetal surgery community quickly realized that relying on evidence for fetal intervention based on retrospective studies of registry data was insufficient. Prospective controlled trials were necessary to determine the efficacy of fetal interventions. In the mid-1980s, UCSF conducted the first trial sponsored by the National Institutes of Health (NIH) to examine open fetal surgical repair for CDH.[14,17] The trial was successfully completed, but concluded that open fetal repair was not beneficial in comparison with standard postnatal care. In addition, patients undergoing fetal surgery had an increased incidence of preterm labor and infection.

Although this trial was logistically difficult, it showed that open fetal repair of CDH defects with liver herniation was not technically feasible, and open fetal surgery to repair diaphragmatic defects was abandoned. However, the conclusions from this trial opened new doors: instead of correcting the anatomic defect, surgeons began trying to reverse CDH-associated pulmonary hypoplasia by temporarily occluding the trachea to stimulate lung growth before birth. Techniques for tracheal occlusion evolved from placing external clips on the trachea during open fetal surgery to deploying a detachable, inflatable balloon device through a single 5-mm uterine port.[18] These developments led to a second prospective, randomized clinical trial at UCSF comparing balloon tracheal occlusion with standard postnatal care for CDH. Although the study showed no difference in outcomes between standard postnatal care and balloon tracheal occlusion (presumably because the potential benefit was offset by the high rate of preterm delivery in the experimental group), it also showed that advances in postnatal care had significantly improved outcomes for patients with severe CDH.

From these early experiences, 3 basic concepts have come to dominate fetal surgery. First, an emphasis has been placed on randomized controlled trials instead of retrospective clinical trials. Next, there has been a move away from anatomic repair of congenital anomalies to physiologic manipulation of the developmental consequences (eg, the shift from in utero repair of the CDH defect to balloon tracheal occlusion to promote lung growth). Finally, there has been a movement toward developing minimally invasive techniques. These overarching principles serve as a guide for the multidisciplinary team of obstetricians, surgeons, perinatologists, and sonologists to promote maternal safety while improving outcomes for patients with fetal anomalies.

By the 1990s, trials for fetal intervention were being performed in many different fetal treatment centers across the world (**Table 1**). In 2005, a cooperative clinical research network, the North American Fetal Therapy Network (NAFTNet), was formed to promote multi-institutional trials in the United States and Canada to study fetal disease, develop prenatal interventions, and improve outcomes. Similarly, the Eurofoetus group was formed in Europe to promote multicenter clinical trials and to foster innovation in fetal medicine.

The Eurofoetus group conducted a nonrandomized trial comparing fetoscopic balloon tracheal occlusion and standard postnatal care in fetuses with severe CDH, which was defined using the observed to expected mean for gestation lung area to head circumference ratio (LHR).[19,20] This study reported that fetoscopic tracheal occlusion increased survival rates from 24% to 49% in left-sided CDH.[20] The group also compared laser ablation with amnioreduction for twin-twin transfusion syndrome, and reported improved survival of at least one twin and fewer neurologic complications with laser ablation.[21] This study was followed by a prospective, randomized multicenter trial in North America for twin-twin transfusion, which did not show statistical significance.[22]

Most recently, the Management of Myelomeningocele Study (MOMS) trial, a multicenter, randomized controlled trial comparing prenatal repair of myelomeningocele (MMC) with postnatal repair, was completed in 2011.[23] Recruitment was terminated early because initial data showed that prenatal repair of MMC decreased rates of ventriculoperitoneal shunt placement for hydrocephalus after birth and improved motor development at 30 months. Although this multicenter trial was difficult to implement,

Table 1
Milestones in fetal therapy

Rhesus disease: IUT	New Zealand	1961
Hysterotomy for fetal vascular access and IUT	Puerto Rico	1964
Respiratory distress syndrome of prematurity: prenatal steroids	London	1972
Fetoscopy: diagnostic	Yale	1974
Experimental pathophysiology (sheep model)	UCSF	1980
Hysterotomy and maternal safety (monkey model)	UCSF	1981
Uropathy: vesicoamniotic shunt	UCSF	1982
Hydrocephalus: ventriculoamniotic shunt	Denver	1982
Uropathy: open fetal surgery	UCSF	1983
IFMSS founded	Santa Barbara	1982
CCAM: resection	UCSF	1984
Intravascular transfusion	London	1985
CDH: open repair	UCSF	1989
Anomalous twin-cord ligation	London	1990
CDH: NIH trial for open repair	UCSF	1990
Aortic valvuloplasty	London	1991
SCT: resection	UCSF	1992
Laser ablation of placental vessels	Milwaukee; London	1995
EXIT procedure for airway obstruction	UCSF	1995
Fetoscopic surgery (Fetendo)	UCSF	1996
XSCID: in utero stem cell transplant	Detroit	1996
Eurofoetus founded	Leuven	1997
CDH: Fetendo clip → balloon	UCSF	1997
Myelomeningocele: open repair	Vanderbilt	1997
CDH: NIH trial for Fetendo balloon	UCSF	1998
Twin reversed-arterial perfusion: radiofrequency ablation	UCSF	1998
Twin reversed-arterial perfusion: cord electrocautery	Leuven	1999
Resection of pericardial teratoma	UCSF	2000
CCAM: prenatal steroid therapy	UCSF	2001
Resection of cervical teratoma	UCSF	2001
CDH: fetoscopic tracheal occlusion (FETO) trial	Leuven; London; Barcelona	2002
Myelomeningocele: NIH trial for open repair	UCSF; CHOP; Vanderbilt	2002
Osteogenesis imperfecta: in utero stem cell transplant	Stockholm	2003
Twin-twin transfusion syndrome: amnioreduction vs laser	Poissy; Eurofoetus	2004
Hypoplastic left heart syndrome: balloon septotomy, valve dilation	Boston	2004
Hypoplastic left heart syndrome: laser atrial septotomy	Tampa	2005
NAFTNet founded	USA and Canada	2005
Amniotic collagen plug	Leuven	2007
CCAM: sclerotherapy	Venezuela; Tampa	2007

Abbreviations: CCAM, congenital cystic adenomatoid formation; CDH, congenital diaphragmatic hernia; CHOP, Children's Hospital of Philadelphia; EXIT, ex utero intrapartum treatment; IFMSS, International Fetal Medicine and Surgery Society; IUT, intrauterine transfusion; NAFTNet, North American Fetal Therapy Network; NIH, National Institutes of Health; SCT, sacrococcygeal teratoma; UCSF, University of California, San Francisco; XSCID, X-linked severe combined immunodeficiency.
Adapted from Jancelewicz T, Harrison MR. A history of fetal surgery. Clin Perinatol 2009;36(2):230; with permission.

Box 1
Basic components of the fetal care team

- Designated team leader
- Care coordinator
- Pediatric cardiologist to perform fetal echocardiogram
- Fetal surgeon: usually a pediatric surgeon or a perinatologist
- Genetic counselor
- Pediatric radiologist to interpret fetal magnetic resonance imaging
- Maternal-fetal medicine specialist
- Neonatologist
- Obstetric anesthetist
- Pediatric anesthetist
- Social worker
- Ultrasonologist

---

it has already had a profound effect on the treatment of MMC, has had an impact on reimbursement standards for fetal intervention, and has defined how fetal surgery centers should be organized and staffed across the United States.

CONSIDERATIONS IN A FETAL TREATMENT PROGRAM

Centers dedicated to fetal treatment require a collaborative team of specialists who are dedicated to continuity of care for both the mother and the fetus. An obstetrician, who is an expert in prenatal diagnosis, amniocentesis, chorionic villus sampling, complications of pregnancy, and family counseling, is important for management of the pregnancy. Pediatric surgeons and neonatologists, who understand the pathophysiology behind neonatal diseases and their treatment after birth, are important

---

Box 2
Participating organizations in guidelines for fetal therapy in myelomeningocele

American Academy of Pediatrics

American College of Obstetricians and Gynecologists

American Institute of Ultrasound in Medicine

American Pediatric Surgical Association

American Society of Anesthesiologists

American Society of Pediatric Neurosurgeons

International Fetal Medicine and Surgery Society

Joint Section of Pediatric Neurosurgery (American Association of Neurological Surgeons/ Congress of Neurological Surgeons)

North American Fetal Therapy Network

Society for Maternal-Fetal Medicine

Spina Bifida Association

for developing a therapeutic plan. The skills of an obstetric sonographer are also invaluable in delineating the fetal anomaly and in guiding diagnostic and therapeutic interventions. Depending on the fetal anomaly, a pediatric cardiologist, neurologist, nephrologist, neurosurgeon, anesthesiologist, or endocrinologist can also be indispensable to the fetal treatment team.

With so many different specialties involved in fetal medicine and fetal surgery, personality conflicts are not uncommon and many questions surface. For instance, who should perform open fetal surgery? Should it be the pediatric surgeon, who has experience repairing complex congenital anomalies in neonates, or the obstetrician, who has experience operating on the gravid uterus? There is currently no specialty that completely encompasses all aspects of care involved in fetal surgery. Therefore, the key to a successful and productive fetal treatment program is a collaborative, multidisciplinary team, which includes an obstetrician, perinatologist, geneticist, sonologist, surgeon, neonatologist, and anesthesiologist, in addition to

---

Box 3
NIH guidelines: development of centers for fetal repair of myelomeningocele

- Fetal MMC repairs should be performed in established fetal therapy centers using a multidisciplinary team approach.

- The fetal surgery team must have experience working together and individual members have a level of expertise in their field.

- The level of fetal surgical technical expertise demanded requires an annual volume of at least 10 cases, including open fetal and EXIT (ex utero intrapartum treatment) procedures.

- The level of technical expertise in fetal MMC repair requires an initial experience of at least 5 cases and an ongoing annual volume of at least 30 MMC cases evaluated for fetal surgery.

- Centers developing new programs must receive guidance and training from established programs and experienced individuals.

- The MOMS protocol should be strictly followed for preoperative, intraoperative, and immediate postoperative care. Modification of the long-term postoperative and delivery care is acceptable in certain circumstances.

- Modifications to the perioperative protocol are only permissible after the results of fetal MMC repair performed by an expanded number of centers have been shown to be consistent with the results obtained in the MOMS trial. Such modifications would, ideally, be developed by means of a series of cooperative trials.

- Ongoing neonatal and pediatric care should be performed in multidisciplinary spina bifida clinics. This can be done at outside centers but must be standardized.

- Counseling should be full disclosure and nondirective in nature. It should also include reproductive implications for future pregnancies.

- A reflective period of at least 24 hours is recommended.

- Short-term and long-term outcomes data from all centers should be kept in a national registry with periodic review.

- Centers performing open MMC repair must maintain a collaborative approach to outcomes reporting and future research, including participating in the collection and evaluation of long-term outcomes data.

- Close links between fetal centers throughout the country and community providers are essential.

Adapted from The MMC Maternal-Fetal Management Task Force. Guidelines for fetal myelomeningocele repair.

experienced support personnel (**Box 1**). These interactions should be formalized with a weekly multidisciplinary meeting, where patients are discussed in depth and plans are formulated among all specialists and personnel involved. Through these weekly interactions, care plans and interventions are mapped with consensus across disciplines.

A close working relationship between perinatal specialists is crucial to success in a fetal treatment program. However, the institution also needs to be adequately equipped to care for fetal patients. Together this requires a high-risk obstetric unit with obstetricians who are available around the clock and have experience delivering patients with a recent hysterotomy, a Level IIIC neonatal intensive care unit, and an environment where research is combined with clinical care. Centers interested in developing a new fetal treatment program should consult existing fetal treatment centers for guidance. In response to the results of the MOMS trial, a multiorganizational task force of representatives from 12 national and international societies (**Box 2**) published guidelines for centers interested in developing fetal intervention programs (**Box 3**). This broadly based document serves as a starting point for individuals interested in starting a fetal intervention program. Because fetal intervention is a new frontier, experience, success, and failure must be critically analyzed and documented to improve patient care and improve understanding.

At UCSF, detailed obstetric and medical histories are reviewed before offering a consultation at the Fetal Treatment Center. Families often elect to travel from across the country for consultations on short notice. Although last-minute flight reservations and housing accommodation are difficult and expensive, these families are eligible for discount travel through programs such as United Airlines' Friendly Skies Program and American Airlines' Miles for Kids. Many fetal treatment centers also offer families accommodation, such as the Ronald McDonald House, to help deflect the costs of travel. The Fetal Treatment Center at UCSF has been fortunate to have a strong institutional commitment to fetal therapy, which was absolutely necessary in the early years when there was little to no insurance or Medicaid reimbursement. Families, who are already burdened by the diagnosis of a fetal anomaly and must prepare for the needs of a sick infant after birth, should not have to assume the financial burden for fetal intervention, especially if it can help deflect health care costs postnatally.

SUMMARY

Over the past 30 years, fetal surgery has evolved into a multidisciplinary, collaborative medical specialty that strives to improve outcomes in patients diagnosed with fetal anomalies. Physicians dedicated to fetal medicine and fetal surgery have formed a cooperative community dedicated to reporting both good and poor outcomes from fetal intervention. Through these collaborations, several multicenter, randomized controlled clinical trials have been successfully completed. Finally, fetal surgery could not have been established as a medical specialty without dedicated physicians, support staff, and institutional support.

REFERENCES

1. DeLorimier AA, Tierney DF, Parker HR. Hypoplastic lungs in fetal lambs with surgically produced congenital diaphragmatic hernia. Surgery 1967;62(1):12–7.
2. Thomasson BH, Esterly JR, Ravitch MM. Morphologic changes in fetal rabbit kidney after intrauterine ureteral ligation. Investig Urol 1970;8(3):261–72.
3. Beck AD. The effect of intra-uterine urinary obstruction upon development of fetal kidney. J Urol 1971;105(6):784–9.

4. Liley AW. Intrauterine transfusion of foetus in haemolytic disease. Br Med J 1963; 2:1107–9.
5. Freda VJ, Adamsons KJ. Exchange transfusion in utero. Report of a case. Obstet Gynecol Surv 1964;19(6):969–71.
6. Asensio SH, Figueroa-Longo JG, Pelegrina IA. Intrauterine exchange transfusion: a new technique. Obstet Gynecol 1968;32(3):350–5.
7. Adamsons K Jr. Fetal surgery. N Engl J Med 1966;275(4):204–6.
8. Harrison MR, Filly RA, Parer JT, et al. Management of the fetus with a urinary-tract malformation. JAMA 1981;246(6):635–9.
9. Harrison MR, Golbus MS, Filly RA. Management of the fetus with a correctable congenital defect. JAMA 1981;246(7):774–7.
10. Adzick NS, Outwater KM, Harrison MR, et al. Correction of congenital diaphragmatic hernia in utero IV. An early gestational fetal lamb model for pulmonary vascular morphometric analysis. J Pediatr Surg 1985;20(6):673–80.
11. Hedrick MH, Estes JM, Sullivan KM, et al. Plug the lung until it grows (plug)— a new method to treat congenital diaphragmatic-hernia in-utero. J Pediatr Surg 1994;29(5):612–7.
12. Deprest JA, Evrard VA, Van Ballaer PP, et al. Tracheoscopic endoluminal plugging using an inflatable device in the fetal lamb model. Eur J Obstet Gynecol Reprod Biol 1998;81(2):165–9.
13. Golbus MS, Harrison MR, Filly RA, et al. In utero treatment of urinary tract obstruction. Am J Obstet Gynecol 1982;142(4):383–8.
14. Clewell WH, Johnson ML, Meier PR, et al. A surgical approach to the treatment of fetal hydrocephalus. N Engl J Med 1982;306(22):1320–5.
15. Harrison MR, Filly RA, Golbus MS, et al. Fetal treatment 1982. N Engl J Med 1982; 307(26):1651–2.
16. Manning FA, Harrison MR, Rodeck C. Catheter shunts for fetal hydronephrosis and hydrocephalus—report of the International Fetal Surgery Registry. N Engl J Med 1986;315(5):336–40.
17. Harrison MR, Adzick NS, Bullard KM, et al. Correction of congenital diaphragmatic hernia in utero VII: a prospective trial. J Pediatr Surg 1997;32(11):1637–42.
18. Harrison MR, Keller RL, Hawgood SB, et al. A randomized trial of fetal endoscopic tracheal occlusion for severe fetal congenital diaphragmatic hernia. N Engl J Med 2003;349(20):1916–24.
19. Deprest J, Gratacos E, Nicolaides KH, et al. Fetoscopic tracheal occlusion (FETO) severe congenital diaphragmatic hernia: evolution of a technique and preliminary results. Ultrasound Obstet Gynecol 2004;24(5):121–6.
20. Jani JC, Nicolaides KH, Gratacós E, et al. Severe diaphragmatic hernia treated by fetal endoscopic tracheal occlusion. Ultrasound Obstet Gynecol 2009;34(3): 304–10.
21. Senat MV, Deprest J, Boulvain M, et al. Endoscopic laser surgery versus serial amnioreduction for severe twin-to-twin transfusion syndrome. N Engl J Med 2004;351(2):136–44.
22. Crombleholme TM, Shera D, Lee H, et al. A prospective, randomized, multicenter trial of amnioreduction vs selective fetoscopic laser photocoagulation for the treatment of severe twin-twin transfusion syndrome. Am J Obstet Gynecol 2007;197(4):396, e1–9.
23. Adzick NS, Thom EA, Spong CY, et al. A randomized trial of prenatal versus postnatal repair of myelomeningocele. N Engl J Med 2011;364(11):993–1004.

Fetal Surgery for Myelomeningocele

Payam Saadai, MD[a],*, Diana L. Farmer, MD, FRCS[b]

KEYWORDS

- Fetal surgery • Hydrocephalus • Myelomeningocele • Neural tube defect • Shunt
- Spina bifida • Ventriculomegaly

KEY POINTS

- Fetal surgery for myelomeningocele is the most common open fetal surgery currently performed, and has been tested in a randomized controlled trial.
- Prenatal repair of myelomeningocele can improve hindbrain herniation and reduce postnatal shunt requirement.
- Distal neurologic function may also be improved in some patients after prenatal repair.
- Fetoscopic approaches to myelomeningocele repair remain a challenge and are an active area of research.

BACKGROUND

Myelomeningocele (MMC) is a congenital neural tube defect that occurs in approximately 1 in 2900 live births in the United States.[1,2] This neurologic anomaly arises from incomplete neural tube closure during early development, resulting in an open spinal canal with exposed neural elements in the form of a flat neural placode. The neural placode then undergoes further traumatic injury in utero. These events form the basis of the two-hit hypothesis of neurologic injury in MMC, with the first hit being the developmental defect itself and the second hit being the additional injury to the exposed neural elements of the spinal cord. In utero intervention to repair the spinal cord does not address the developmental defect, but can ameliorate the subsequent trauma associated with the second hit.

Disclosure statement: Diana L. Farmer is a principal investigator on the Management of Myelomeningocele Study (MOMS) and received NIH funding for this work (grant no. NICHD 3U10 HD041669). The authors have no other relevant affiliations or financial involvement with any organization or entity with a financial interest in or financial conflict with the subject matter or materials discussed in the article apart from those disclosed.

[a] Division of Pediatric Surgery, Department of Surgery, Fetal Treatment Center, University of California, San Francisco, 513 Parnassus Avenue, HSW 16-01, Box 0570, San Francisco, CA 94143-0570, USA; [b] Division of Pediatric Surgery, Department of Surgery, UC Davis School of Medicine, UC Davis Children's Hospital, UC Davis Health System, 2221 Stockton Boulevard, Suite 3112, Sacramento, CA 95817, USA
* Corresponding author.
E-mail address: payam.saadai@ucsfmedctr.org

Clin Perinatol 39 (2012) 279–288
doi:10.1016/j.clp.2012.04.003 **perinatology.theclinics.com**

The exact etiology of MMC is unknown, but its origin is likely multifactorial. Nutritional, environmental, and genetic factors have all been implicated in the pathogenesis of MMC. Folate deficiency in mothers is associated with an increased incidence of neural tube defects. Folate supplementation can decrease the risk of MMC in the pregnancy by as much as 50%, but it has not eradicated the anomaly.[3] Environmental exposure to toxins and drugs has been implicated in the development of neural tube defects. In addition, genetic abnormalities may have a role in some patients, as seen in patients with in PAX3 mutation in Waardenburg syndrome for example.

Patients with MMC can display a broad array of clinical findings depending on the severity of their neurologic defect. Most infants survive the neonatal period without significant morbidity; however, up to 30% of patients die before adulthood because of respiratory, urinary, or central nervous system complications. Long-term morbidity and mortality is related both to neurologic damage from the spinal cord lesion itself and to brain abnormalities from leakage of cerebrospinal fluid.[4] Continued leakage of cerebrospinal fluid is thought to lead to an intercerebral pressure gradient, resulting in a hindbrain herniation known as Arnold-Chiari II malformation. Virtually all newborns with MMC have a Chiari malformation and more than 90% will develop hydrocephalus, requiring ventriculoperitoneal (VP) shunting. The spinal level of the defect determines the degree of motor and somatosensory deficit. In addition, these patients often have dysfunction of bladder and bowel control, as well as loss of sexual function that manifests in adolescence and early adulthood.[5]

RATIONALE FOR FETAL REPAIR OF MMC

The rationale for fetal repair of MMC targets the second hit of the two-hit hypothesis.[6,7] By limiting in utero damage to the exposed spinal cord and preventing continued leakage of cerebrospinal fluid, in utero coverage of the spinal defect could potentially normalize the intercerebral gradient and lead to improved neurologic outcomes. Several observations in both humans and animals support the two-hit hypothesis. First, early prenatal ultrasonographic examination of human fetuses with MMC has demonstrated normal hindlimb movement.[8] This finding suggests a later loss of function attributable to in utero injury to the spinal cord. Second, postmortem analysis of stillborn and aborted fetuses with MMC has suggested recent in utero injury to the exposed neural placode.[6] Third, patients with milder forms of neural tube defects whereby abnormal neural elements remain covered with skin or a membrane have more normal neural development than those patients with MMC.[9] Finally, observations in mice with neural tube defects have demonstrated normal early anatomy and function, which is then progressively lost in utero.[10]

ANIMAL MODELS

Animal models were developed to study the natural history of MMC and potential fetal interventions before attempting fetal MMC repair in humans. Surgical models in rodent, rabbit, sheep, and nonhuman primates share a similar phenotype to that found in human MMC: paraplegia, extremity deformity, urinary and bowel dysfunction, hydrocephalus, and the Chiari malformation. Prenatal closure of these surgically created defects has produced improvement in motor function and urinary function, and reversal of the Chiari malformation, with normal or near-normal hindbrain development and morphology. Several animal models have demonstrated that the Chiari malformation occurs with surgically created myelomeningocele and, more importantly, that it can be reversed after in utero repair.[11–15] Further animal studies have also demonstrated improved distal neurologic function after in utero repair of surgically created MMC. In a rabbit model of fetal MMC repair, neurologic function was improved after birth, as measured by somatosensory-evoked potentials.[16] In studies examining anal sphincter development in the sheep model, histologic examination of rectum and anal sphincter muscles revealed preservation of longitudinal muscles in the sphincter complex and the submucosal nerve plexus in lambs that had undergone fetal repair.[17,18]

EARLY HUMAN EXPERIENCE
Fetoscopic Repair

Before the advent of prenatal repair for MMC, human fetal surgery had been reserved for situations whereby there would be expected perinatal mortality. This approach was adopted to maximize potential benefit in the fetus while minimizing risk and morbidity to the mother. Fetal diseases for which prenatal intervention was considered included severe obstructive uropathies, congenital diaphragmatic hernia, placental anomalies such as twin-twin transfusion syndrome, and nonimmune hydrops secondary to an anatomic defect (eg, sacrococcygeal teratoma, congenital cystic adenoid malformation). MMC was the first nonlethal fetal malformation treated with human in utero surgery.

In an attempt to minimize maternal morbidity, early human fetal MMC repairs were approached fetoscopically.[19–21] This technique was independently attempted at the Vanderbilt University Medical Center and at the University of California, San Francisco (UCSF). The Vanderbilt group reported 4 fetoscopic repairs via maternal laparotomy and a 3-port technique for in utero access. The amniotic fluid was replaced with carbon dioxide and the defects were covered with a maternal skin graft. Two of 4 fetuses survived to birth; both survivors required reoperation postnatally because no evidence of the skin graft was found at birth.

The UCSF group reported 3 attempts at fetoscopic MMC repair, only 1 of which was successfully closed fetoscopically. In this patient the MMC defect was closed with a decellularized dermal matrix patch; however, at birth the repair was incomplete and required an additional operation to close the defect. The 2 other attempts at fetoscopic repair were converted to open fetal repair because of technical difficulties. Fetoscopic repair would eventually be largely abandoned in favor of open fetal repair, which was technically easier to complete despite its increased maternal morbidity.

Open Repair

After these early attempts at minimally invasive repair, fetal surgeons began performing open fetal MMC repair (**Fig. 1**). The Vanderbilt group was the first to report its results in 1999, and concluded that the open repair method was superior to the fetoscopic method. This group also found that hindbrain herniation was improved in MMC patients who had undergone fetal surgical repair and that the need for VP shunting was significantly lower in these patients: 59% versus 91% in historical controls.[22] These data were limited by their small sample size and the lack of a standardized protocol for postnatal VP shunt placement. A follow-up study with subset analysis demonstrated that repair earlier in gestation, lower-level lesions, and smaller ventricles before repair were all associated with a lower VP shunt rate.[23,24]

Concurrently, the group at the Children's Hospital of Philadelphia (CHOP) confirmed the findings of reversal of hindbrain herniation and improvement in the Chiari malformation in patients who had undergone open fetal repair.[25] These findings were corroborated with studies of head biometry in prenatal and postnatal magnetic resonance imaging scans.[26] Decreased shunt rates and less ventriculomegaly were also reported, further reinforcing the findings at Vanderbilt.[27]

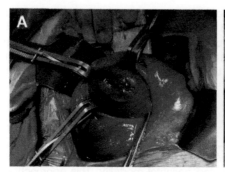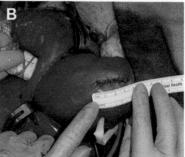

Fig. 1. Open fetal repair of myelomeningocele. (*A*) Myelomeningocele defect before repair. (*B*) Final skin closure of a myelomeningocele defect.

Neurologic Function

At all 3 centers, immediate results did not reveal significant improvement in neurologic function or hindlimb movement with fetal repair. Follow-up data were mixed. At UCSF, only 2 of 9 survivors had functional improvement greater than 2 spinal levels above the MMC lesion. Neurologic function correlated well with the level of the spinal lesion in the remainder of patients.[21] The Vanderbilt group initially compared the neurologic outcomes of 26 patients who had undergone fetal MMC repair with historical controls and found no improvement.[28] Their cohort was later compared with matched controls at the University of Alabama, Birmingham, and again they found no improvement in neurologic function.[29] By contrast, the CHOP group examined 54 patients who had fetal MMC repair and found that 57% had neurologic function better than what was predicted from the level of their spinal defect.[30] Their median follow-up was 66 months and ranged from 36 to 133 months. Factors that were associated with a lower likelihood of independent ambulation included higher-level lesions and presence of a clubfoot deformity.

Maternal Morbidity

Open fetal surgery places the healthy mother at risk for significant operative and postoperative complications. Two early studies suggested that maternal morbidity was low and that fertility after fetal surgery was preserved.[31,32] However, the Vanderbilt data revealed more serious maternal morbidity: intraoperative placenta abruption, uterine dehiscence, and small bowel obstruction.[33] Uterine dehiscence and rupture are particularly notable because these risks remain present for any subsequent pregnancies.

Prematurity

Two reports were published from the Vanderbilt group regarding prematurity in neonates who underwent fetal repair of MMC. The first report analyzed whether repair before 25 weeks' gestation affected gestational age at birth, and found that the degree of prematurity was independent of the gestational age at fetal repair.[34] A follow-up study compared the complication rate of premature infants who had fetal repair of MMC with that of controls matched for gestational age, sex, birth weight, antenatal steroid use, and mode of delivery, and found no significant difference in the incidence of morbidity associated with prematurity.[35]

Urologic Function

Studies of urologic outcome in infants who underwent prenatal closure of MMC have to date demonstrated no improvement in urologic function. The Vanderbilt group examined 16 patients with a mean age of 6.5 months and compared urodynamic studies with those from historical controls. Similar results between the two groups were found.[36] The UCSF group examined 6 patients who had fetal MMC repair and also found no significant urologic improvement.[37]

THE MANAGEMENT OF MYELOMENINGOCELE STUDY

From these early reported case series, it was unclear whether prenatal repair of MMC was beneficial when compared with standard postnatal therapy, as no controlled comparisons had been made. To address this question, in 2003 CHOP, Vanderbilt, and UCSF began collaboration on a National Institutes of Health–sponsored prospective randomized controlled trial (Management of Myelomeningocele Study, or MOMS) comparing prenatal MMC repair with postnatal repair.[38] Inclusion and exclusion criteria for the trial are listed in **Box 1**.

There were 2 primary research questions in this trial. The first was whether fetal surgery for MMC improved outcomes as measured by death or the need for a VP shunt within the first year of life. The second question was whether prenatal repair of MMC improved neurologic function at 30 months of age as predicted by the spinal level of the lesion. Secondary research questions included whether the Chiari malformation was improved, whether neuromotor outcome was improved at 12 and 30 months of age, and the long-term psychological and reproductive consequences for the parents.

Outcomes

In 2011, enrollment in the MOMS trial was stopped early because of statistical evidence of benefit in the prenatal surgery group after the enrollment of 183 of a planned 200 patients. Initial analysis of the first 158 patients confirmed that fetal surgery for MMC had decreased the need for postnatal VP shunting in approximately one-third of infants by 12 months (**Table 1**). The proportion of infants who had no evidence of hindbrain herniation was significantly higher in the prenatal surgery group, and the proportion of infants who had moderate or severe hindbrain herniation was significantly reduced. The second primary outcome, neurologic function as assessed by a score derived from mental and motor development at 30 months, was also significantly improved in the prenatal surgery group. In addition, several secondary outcomes were improved. Most notably, the percentage of patients able to independently ambulate at 30 months increased from 21% to 42% after prenatal repair compared with postnatal surgery, supporting the theory that distal neurologic function can also be improved by in utero closure.

There were no maternal deaths and 2 perinatal deaths in each group, suggesting that mortality was comparable between groups. Prenatal surgery was associated with higher rates of preterm birth, intraoperative complications, uterine-scar defects, and higher rates of maternal transfusion at delivery, all of which are known complications of open fetal surgery. Although enrollment into the MOMS trial has ended, long-term follow-up and analysis is ongoing. In addition, a new study (MOMS II) will follow up the neurologic outcome of these patients into later childhood.

NEW DIRECTIONS

To augment the still limited neurologic function recovered by fetal MMC repair, novel regenerative medicine techniques are being actively studied in research laboratories. One study of murine neural stem cells applied to the MMC defect during fetal repair in sheep showed qualitative improvements in hindlimb movement in the animals that

---

Box 1
Inclusion and exclusion criteria for the Management of Myelomeningocele Study

Inclusion Criteria:

1. Myelomeningocele at level T1 through S1 with hindbrain herniation

2. Maternal age 18 years or older

3. Gestational age at randomization of 19^0 to 25^6 weeks

4. Normal karyotype

Exclusion Criteria:

1. Nonresident of the United States

2. Nonsingleton pregnancy

3. Insulin-dependent pregestational diabetes

4. Fetal anomaly not related to MMC

5. Kyphosis in the fetus of 30° or greater

6. Current or planned cerclage or documented history of incompetent cervix

7. Short cervix (<20 mm)

8. Placenta previa or placental abruption

9. Body mass index 35 kg/m^2 or greater

10. Previous spontaneous delivery before 37 weeks' gestation

11. Maternal-fetal Rh isoimmunization, Kell sensitization, or neonatal alloimmune thrombocytopenia

12. Maternal human immunodeficiency virus or hepatitis B status positive

13. Known hepatitis C positivity

14. Uterine anomaly such as large or multiple fibroids or Müllerian duct abnormality

15. Other maternal medical condition that is a contraindication to surgery or general anesthesia

16. Patient does not have a support person

17. Inability to comply with travel and follow-up requirements

18. Patient does not meet other psychosocial criteria to handle the implications of the trial

19. Participation in another intervention study that influences maternal and fetal morbidity and mortality or participation in this trial during a previous pregnancy

20. Maternal hypertension that would increase the risk of preeclampsia or preterm delivery

---

received stem cells.[39] The neural stem cells survived and engrafted, and they appeared to be more concentrated at areas of greatest damage, suggesting that they may "home in" on the most injured areas. On further histologic analysis, the engrafted neural stem cells were found to remain in a largely undifferentiated state, possibly suggesting a neurotrophic secretory or chaperone-like role for these cells. Other groups are exploring the use of biomaterials such as gelatin microspheres and nanofibrous scaffolds as a means to maximize the unique benefits of prenatal MMC closure.[40,41] This research is preliminary, but supports further study on the benefits of a multifaceted approach to MMC repair. Because of the maternal morbidity of open fetal surgery, less invasive methods of fetal MMC treatment continue to be investigated.[42,43] In addition, surgical experiments in fetal sheep have demonstrated

Table 1
Summary of select outcomes from the Management of Myelomeningocele Study randomized controlled trial

	Prenatal Surgery (N = 78)	Postnatal Surgery (N = 80)	Relative Risk (95% CI)	P Value
Primary Outcomes				
Primary outcome at 12 months[a]	53 (68%)	78 (98%)	0.70 (0.58–0.84)	<.001
Primary outcome at 30 months[b]	148.6 ± 57.5 (SD)	122.6 ± 57.2 (SD)	—	.007
Secondary Outcomes				
Hindbrain herniation (12 months)	45/70 (64%)	66/69 (96%)	0.67 (0.56–0.81)	<.001
Shunt placement (12 months)	31 (40%)	66 (82%)	0.48 (0.36–0.64)	<.001
Walking independently (30 months)	26/62 (42%)	14/67 (21%)	2.01 (1.16–3.48)	.01

Abbreviation: CI, confidence interval.
[a] Based on incidence of fetal or neonatal death or need for shunt placement by 12 months.
[b] Composite score based on Bayley Mental Developmental Index and the difference between observed and expected motor function at age 30 months. Higher values indicate better function.

the feasibility of robot-assisted closure of MMC defects.[44] Given the push toward fetoscopic closure, it is likely that a less invasive fetal MMC technique will become accepted in the near future.

SUMMARY

Myelomeningocele is a devastating disability with significant morbidity and mortality within the first few decades of life. MMC was the first nonlethal disease to be considered and studied for fetal surgery. The recently completed MOMS trial has shown that fetal repair for MMC can improve hydrocephalus and hindbrain herniation associated with the Arnold-Chiari II malformation, can reduce the need for VP shunting, and may improve distal neurologic function in some patients. Potential improvements in outcome must be balanced with the safety and well-being of the mother in addition to that of the unborn patient. Further follow-up will determine the long-term benefit of fetal MMC repair.

REFERENCES

1. Canfield MA, Honein MA, Yuskiv N, et al. National estimates and race/ethnic-specific variation of selected birth defects in the United States, 1999-2001. Birth Defects Res A Clin Mol Teratol 2006;76(11):747–56.
2. Boulet SL, Yang Q, Mai C, et al. Trends in the postfortification prevalence of spina bifida and anencephaly in the United States. Birth Defects Res A Clin Mol Teratol 2008;82:527–32.
3. De Wals P, Tairou F, Van Allen MI, et al. Reduction in neural-tube defects after folic acid fortification in Canada. N Engl J Med 2007;357(2):135–42.
4. Steinbok P, Irvine B, Cochrane DD, et al. Long-term outcome and complications of children born with meningomyelocele. Childs Nerv Syst 1992;8(2):92–6.

5. Woodhouse CRJ. Myelomeningocele: neglected aspects. Pediatr Nephrol 2008; 23:1223–31.
6. Hutchins GM, Meuli M, Meuli-Simmen C, et al. Acquired spinal cord injury in human fetuses with myelomeningocele. Pediatr Pathol Lab Med 1996;16(5): 701–12.
7. Heffez DS, Aryanpur J, Hutchins GM, et al. The paralysis associated with myelomeningocele: clinical and experimental data implicating a preventable spinal cord injury. Neurosurgery 1990;26(6):987–92.
8. Korenromp MJ, van Gool JD, Bruinese HW, et al. Early fetal leg movements in myelomeningocele. Lancet 1986;1(8486):917–8.
9. Oya N, Suzuki Y, Tanemura M, et al. Detection of skin over cysts with spina bifida may be useful not only for preventing neurological damage during labor but also for predicting fetal prognosis. Fetal Diagn Ther 2000;15(3):156–9.
10. Stiefel D, Copp AJ, Meuli M. Fetal spina bifida in a mouse model: loss of neural function in utero. J Neurosurg 2007;106(Suppl 3):213–21.
11. Pedreira DA, Sanchez e Oliveira Rde C, Valente PR, et al. Validation of the ovine fetus as an experimental model for the human myelomeningocele defect. Acta Cir Bras 2007;22(3):168–73.
12. von Koch CS, Compagnone N, Hirose S, et al. Myelomeningocele: characterization of a surgically induced sheep model and its central nervous system similarities and differences to the human disease. Am J Obstet Gynecol 2005;193(4): 1456–62.
13. Weber Guimaraes Barreto M, Ferro MM, Guimaraes Bittencourt D, et al. Arnold-Chiari in a fetal rat model of dysraphism. Fetal Diagn Ther 2005;20(5):437–41.
14. Paek BW, Farmer DL, Wilkinson CC, et al. Hindbrain herniation develops in surgically created myelomeningocele but is absent after repair in fetal lambs. Am J Obstet Gynecol 2000;183(5):1119–23.
15. Galvan-Montano A, Cardenas-Lailson E, Hernandez-Godinez B, et al. [Development of an animal model of myelomeningocele and options for prenatal treatment in Macaca mulatta]. Cir Cir 2007;75(5):357–62 [in Spanish].
16. Julia V, Sancho MA, Albert A, et al. Prenatal covering of the spinal cord decreases neurologic sequelae in a myelomeningocele model. J Pediatr Surg 2006;41(6): 1125–9.
17. Yoshizawa J, Sbragia L, Paek BW, et al. Fetal surgery for repair of myelomeningocele allows normal development of the rectum in sheep. Pediatr Surg Int 2003;19(3):162–6.
18. Yoshizawa J, Sbragia L, Paek BW, et al. Fetal surgery for repair of myelomeningocele allows normal development of anal sphincter muscles in sheep. Pediatr Surg Int 2004;20(1):14–8.
19. Bruner JP, Richards WO, Tulipan NB, et al. Endoscopic coverage of fetal myelomeningocele in utero. Am J Obstet Gynecol 1999;180(1 Pt 1):153–8.
20. Bruner JP, Tulipan NB, Richards WO, et al. In utero repair of myelomeningocele: a comparison of endoscopy and hysterotomy. Fetal Diagn Ther 2000;15(2):83–8.
21. Farmer DL, von Koch CS, Peacock WJ, et al. In utero repair of myelomeningocele: experimental pathophysiology, initial clinical experience, and outcomes. Arch Surg 2003;138(8):872–8.
22. Bruner JP, Tulipan N, Paschall RL, et al. Fetal surgery for myelomeningocele and the incidence of shunt-dependent hydrocephalus. JAMA 1999;282(19):1819–25.
23. Tulipan N, Sutton LN, Bruner JP, et al. The effect of intrauterine myelomeningocele repair on the incidence of shunt-dependent hydrocephalus. Pediatr Neurosurg 2003;38(1):27–33.

24. Bruner JP, Tulipan N, Reed G, et al. Intrauterine repair of spina bifida: preoperative predictors of shunt-dependent hydrocephalus. Am J Obstet Gynecol 2004; 190(5):1305–12.
25. Sutton LN, Adzick NS, Bilaniuk LT, et al. Improvement in hindbrain herniation demonstrated by serial fetal magnetic resonance imaging following fetal surgery for myelomeningocele. JAMA 1999;282(19):1826–31.
26. Danzer E, Johnson MP, Bebbington M, et al. Fetal head biometry assessed by fetal magnetic resonance imaging following in utero myelomeningocele repair. Fetal Diagn Ther 2007;22(1):1–6.
27. Johnson MP, Sutton LN, Rintoul N, et al. Fetal myelomeningocele repair: short-term clinical outcomes. Am J Obstet Gynecol 2003;189(2):482–7.
28. Tulipan N, Bruner JP, Hernanz-Schulman M, et al. Effect of intrauterine myelomeningocele repair on central nervous system structure and function. Pediatr Neurosurg 1999;31(4):183–8.
29. Tubbs RS, Chambers MR, Smyth MD, et al. Late gestational intrauterine myelomeningocele repair does not improve lower extremity function. Pediatr Neurosurg 2003;38(3):128–32.
30. Tulipan N, Bruner JP. Myelomeningocele repair in utero: a report of 3 cases. Pediatr Neurosurg 1998;28(4):177–80.
31. Farrell JA, Albanese CT, Jennings RW, et al. Maternal fertility is not affected by fetal surgery. Fetal Diagn Ther 1999;14(3):190–2.
32. Danzer E, Gerdes M, Bebbington MW, et al. Lower extremity neuromotor function and short-term ambulatory potential following in utero myelomeningocele surgery. Fetal Diagn Ther 2009;25(1):47–53.
33. Longaker MT, Golbus MS, Filly RA, et al. Maternal outcome after open fetal surgery. A review of the first 17 human cases. JAMA 1991;265(6):737–41.
34. Hamdan AH, Walsh W, Heddings A, et al. Gestational age at intrauterine myelomeningocele repair does not influence the risk of prematurity. Fetal Diagn Ther 2002;17(2):66–8.
35. Hamdan AH, Walsh W, Bruner JP, et al. Intrauterine myelomeningocele repair: effect on short-term complications of prematurity. Fetal Diagn Ther 2004;19(1):83–6.
36. Holzbeierlein J, Pope JI, Adams MC, et al. The urodynamic profile of myelodysplasia in childhood with spinal closure during gestation. J Urol 2000;164(4): 1336–9.
37. Holmes NM, Nguyen HT, Harrison MR, et al. Fetal intervention for myelomeningocele: effect on postnatal bladder function. J Urol 2001;166(6):2383–6.
38. Adzick NS, Thom EA, Spong CY, et al. A randomized trial of prenatal versus postnatal repair of myelomeningocele. N Engl J Med 2011;364(11):993–1004.
39. Fauza DO, Jennings RW, Teng YD, et al. Neural stem cell delivery to the spinal cord in an ovine model of fetal surgery for spina bifida. Surgery 2008;144(3): 367–73.
40. Saadai P, Nout YS, Encinas J, et al. Prenatal repair of myelomeningocele with aligned nanofibrous scaffolds—a pilot study in sheep. J Pediatr Surg 2011;46: 2279–83.
41. Watanabe M, Li H, Roybal J, et al. A tissue engineering approach for prenatal closure of myelomeningocele: comparison of gelatin sponge and microsphere scaffolds and bioactive protein coatings. Tissue Eng Part A 2011;17(7-8): 1099–110.
42. Pedreira DA, Oliveira RC, Valente PR, et al. Gasless fetoscopy: a new approach to endoscopic closure of a lumbar skin defect in fetal sheep. Fetal Diagn Ther 2008;23(4):293–8.

43. Kohl T, Hartlage MG, Kiehitz D, et al. Percutaneous fetoscopic patch coverage of experimental lumbosacral full-thickness skin lesions in sheep. Surg Endosc 2003; 17(8):1218–23.
44. Aaronson OS, Tulipan NB, Cywes R, et al. Robot-assisted endoscopic intrauterine myelomeningocele repair: a feasibility study. Pediatr Neurosurg 2002;36(2):85–9.

Advances in Prenatal Diagnosis and Treatment of Congenital Diaphragmatic Hernia

Eveline H. Shue, MD[a], Doug Miniati, MD[a], Hanmin Lee, MD[b],*

KEYWORDS

- Congenital diaphragmatic hernia • Pulmonary hypoplasia • Pulmonary hypertension
- Lung/head ratio • Liver herniation • EXIT procedure • Tracheal occlusion
- Fetal breathing

KEY POINTS

- The presence or absence of liver herniation and quantification of the lung-to-head ratio are the most accurate prenatal prognostic indicators of survival for fetuses with congenital diaphragmatic hernia.
- Whereas open fetal CDH repair has been abandoned, fetal endoscopic balloon tracheal occlusion has been developed to promote lung growth for severe CDH.
- Tracheal occlusion increases lung volume, DNA, protein, and alveolar surface area, and also decreases pulmonary arteriolar medial wall thickness and muscularization.
- Although significant improvements in lung function have yet to be shown in humans, reversible or dynamic tracheal occlusion holds promise for appropriately selected fetuses with severe CDH.

INTRODUCTION

Congenital diaphragmatic hernia (CDH) is a common birth anomaly, with an incidence of 1 in 2400 newborn infants.[1] The true incidence of CDH is likely higher, because those with severe defects often abort spontaneously, die in utero, or die shortly after birth.[2] Before 10 weeks' gestation, abdominal viscera herniate through a diaphragmatic defect into the thoracic cavity during fetal development and compress the developing lung, causing lung hypoplasia. However, studies in the nitrofen rodent model of CDH suggest that the pathophysiology behind CDH may be more complex than simple mechanical compression of the developing lung. In the nitrofen rodent model of CDH, pulmonary hypoplasia occurs primarily before development of the diaphragmatic hernia and even in the absence of a diaphragmatic hernia phenotype.

[a] Division of Pediatric Surgery, Department of Surgery, Fetal Treatment Center University of California, San Francisco, 513 Parnassus Avenue, HSW-1601, San Francisco, CA 94143-0570, USA; [b] Division of Pediatric Surgery, Fetal Treatment Center, UCSF Benioff Children's Hospital, 513 Parnassus Avenue, HSW 1601, San Francisco, CA 94143, USA
* Corresponding author.
E-mail address: hanmin.lee@ucsfmedctr.org

Clin Perinatol 39 (2012) 289–300
doi:10.1016/j.clp.2012.04.005   perinatology.theclinics.com
0095-5108/12/$ – see front matter © 2012 Elsevier Inc. All rights reserved.

Pulmonary hypoplasia is further exacerbated by the presence of a diaphragmatic hernia and abdominal contents in the thorax. This model suggests that the pathophysiology behind CDH is multifactorial, and possibly a result of a combination of environmental, teratogenic, and genetic factors. Regardless, pulmonary hypoplasia and pulmonary hypertension lead to persistent fetal circulation and respiratory failure, and remain the main determinants of survival in CDH.

Fetuses with congenital high airway obstruction or laryngeal atresia have hyperplastic lungs at birth, and therefore, temporary tracheal occlusion was developed to promote lung growth for severe CDH. There is a wide spectrum of severity in CDH, which seems to be related to the timing and amount of herniated viscera.[3,4] Some infants with a small diaphragmatic defect and mild lung hypoplasia do well with standard postnatal care, but those with severe lung hypoplasia, pulmonary vascular hypoplasia, and pulmonary hypertension often die in utero or in the neonatal period before transport to a tertiary care center. Infants with severe CDH have a dismal prognosis, with a mortality of 75%.[5] Prognostic factors, such as lung/head ratio (LHR) and the absence or presence of liver herniation, have been described in an attempt to identify those with severe CDH who would benefit from fetal tracheal occlusion. The goal of fetal intervention in CDH is to promote lung growth before birth to improve postnatal gas exchange. Simultaneously, advances in postnatal care using strategies such as gentle ventilation and permissive hypercapnia optimize the available lung function, but mortality from CDH still remains approximately 30%. This article reviews advances in prenatal diagnosis of CDH, the experimental basis for tracheal occlusion, and its translation into human trials in the United States and Europe.

Natural History of CDH and Prenatal Prognosis

The natural history of CDH depends on the severity of disease; retrospective studies have reported that survival ranges from 20% to 76% at tertiary centers that offer extracorporeal membrane oxygenation (ECMO).[6,7] With advances in ultrasound technology, most cases of CDH are now diagnosed prenatally. To improve outcomes in CDH, it is necessary to identify the natural history and stratify patients into those with mild disease who would survive with standard postnatal care and those with severe disease who would normally be unsalvageable. A prospective study of 83 fetuses with isolated CDH before 24 weeks' gestation performed at the University of California, San Francisco (UCSF) between 1989 and 1993 showed a mortality of 58%.[4] Forty-eight patients did not survive: 7 died in utero, 4 were too premature for ECMO, 16 died of respiratory distress before ECMO could be initiated, and 21 died despite management with ECMO. The discrepancy in mortality between different centers likely represents the hidden mortality of CDH. Survival of infants at tertiary care centers automatically selects for patients who survive birth, resuscitation, and transport from an outside facility, and therefore underestimates the true mortality associated with CDH. Studies that evaluate outcome based on postnatal diagnosis of CDH fail to account for fetuses with intrauterine fetal demise and the neonates with early postnatal death who do not undergo an autopsy to identify the cause. Therefore, prenatal diagnosis and prognostic indicators are important to accurately counsel families and identify patients with severe disease who may benefit from fetal intervention.

Several studies have identified indicators of poor outcome, including gestational age at diagnosis,[8] polyhydramnios,[6] an intrathoracic stomach,[9,10] and cardiac ventricular disproportion.[11] However, sonographic evaluation of the LHR and the presence or absence of liver herniation (liver up vs liver down) are the most reliable prognostic indicators that have been identified. Studies show that 42% to 53% of patients with liver up require ECMO, whereas only 0% to 19% of patients with liver down require ECMO.[12,13] In addition, survival in patients with liver up is reported between 19% and 56% whereas survival in patients with liver down ranges from 76% to 100%.[8,12–14]

LHR was first described as the sonographic evaluation of the ratio between the two-dimensional area of the right lung at the level of the atria and the head circumference for left-sided, liver-up CDH in fetuses at or before 25 weeks' gestation.[8] In this study, there were no survivors with an LHR less than 0.6. Fetuses with an LHR between 0.6 and 1.35 had a survival of 61%, and those with an LHR greater than 1.4 had a survival of 100%. In another study, 184 fetuses with isolated left-sided, liver-up CDH had an LHR measured between 22 and 28 weeks of gestation and were followed postnatally for 3 months in a multicenter study associated with the antenatal CDH registry.[14] This study showed that in fetuses with intrathoracic liver herniation and a left-sided CDH, LHR determination between 22 and 28 weeks of gestation is a useful predictor of survival. In contrast, a retrospective study was published disputing the usefulness of LHR as a prognostic indicator of outcome in CDH.[15] Although this small study of 28 patients at a single center did not find a significant difference in survival between those with an LHR less than 1.0 (73% survival) and those with LHR greater than 1.0 (94% survival), this study included patients without liver herniation. The trend toward improved survival in patients with LHR less than 1.0 is likely to be significant in a larger population.

Although LHR is a useful predictor of survival in fetuses with intrathoracic liver herniation up to 28 weeks' gestation, LHR increases exponentially with gestational age.[16] The observed to expected LHR (o/e LHR) was developed by the Antenatal CDH Registry Group, which normalizes LHR to expected lung volumes at gestational age.[17] The investigators report that o/e LHR in normal infants was 100% for both the right and left lung. However, an analysis of 354 infants with CDH between 18 and 38 weeks' gestation showed an average o/e LHR of 39%. Fetuses with an o/e LHR less than 15% had virtually no chance of survival (**Table 1**).[18] Those with an o/e LHR between 15% and 25% have a predicted survival of 20%. Fetuses with an o/e LHR between 26% and 35% irrespective of liver position and those with an o/e LHR between 36% and 45% with liver-up CDH have a predicted survival of 30–60%. Fetuses with an o/e LHR between 36% and 45% with liver-down CDH or an o/e LHR greater than 45% have a predicted survival greater than 75%. This study also examined outcomes in 25 fetuses with right-sided CDH and determined that there were no survivors with an o/e LHR less than 45%.

LHR was developed as a measurement of pulmonary hypoplasia in left-sided CDH to estimate the amount of residual lung tissue. Since the first description of LHR, advances in imaging techniques, including single-shot fast spin echo, have resulted in high-quality magnetic resonance imaging (MRI) that reduces artifact generated by fetal motion. Reports evaluating pulmonary hypoplasia using fetal MRI first

Table 1
Predicted survival (%) based on o/e LHR in prenatally diagnosed CDH

o/e LHR	Liver Up	Liver Down	Survival
<15	—	—	0
15–25	—	—	20
26–35	—	—	36–60
36–45	30–60	>75	—
>45	—	—	>75

emerged in 2001. One study evaluated the ratio of total lung volume to expected lung volume for gestational age in 11 fetuses with left-sided CDH before 27 weeks' gestation and found that infants with a relative lung volume of less than 40% had a mortality of 75%.[19] The correlation between relative lung volume and LHR measured by ultrasonography was significant as well ($R = 0.78$, $P<.001$). In a separate retrospective study of 44 patients at a single institution who underwent fetal MRI between 32 and 34 weeks' gestation, patients with a total lung volume greater than 40 cm³ had a survival of 90% and only 10% required ECMO. In contrast, fetuses with a total lung volume less than 20 cm³ had a survival of 35% and 86% required ECMO.[20] Multiple studies report the use of fetal MRI to measure total lung volume, LHR, or volume of herniated liver to predict neonatal outcome[20–22] and have concluded that relative lung volume is predictive of survival in CDH. However, these studies are all performed at different gestational ages, and there has been no consensus on the threshold for poor prognosis. Although fetal MRI is useful, especially in late gestation when the opportunity to calculate LHR has passed, it has not replaced ultrasonography as a first-line screening technique because ultrasonography is faster and more cost-effective.

Stratification of severity of CDH by LHR has been validated in left-sided CDH with liver herniation.[8] Identification of liver position and LHR as prognostic indicators for outcomes in CDH allows clinicians to counsel expectant families, anticipate the need for ECMO after birth, and identify patients who are unlikely to survive without fetal intervention. Patients without liver herniation and an LHR greater than 1.4 have a favorable prognosis and therefore are not usually offered fetal intervention because of the additional risks of infection, preterm labor, and preterm delivery. Advances in postnatal care, including high-frequency oscillatory ventilation and permissive hypercapnia, have increased survival and improved morbidity in patients with an LHR between 1 and 1.4.[23] However, patients with intrathoracic liver herniation and an LHR less than 1.0 have a high mortality and morbidity, and experimental therapy such as prenatal temporary tracheal occlusion may be recommended to improve outcome.

REVERSING CDH-INDUCED LUNG HYPOPLASIA

To determine if CDH-induced pulmonary hypoplasia could be reversed in utero, Harrison and colleagues[24] inflated silicone balloons in the left hemithorax of fetal lambs to simulate compression of the developing lung by abdominal viscera between gestational day 100 and 145. Despite full resuscitation, 4 lambs born at term gestation by cesarean delivery died, and pathologic examination showed severe lung hypoplasia. A subsequent study showed decreased lung compliance and decreased cross-sectional area of the pulmonary vascular bed.[25] However, when these silicone balloons were deflated at 120 days' gestation, lambs that were born at term gestation survived, had improved lung compliance, and increased pulmonary vasculature.[26] These results were encouraging, and in utero simulated repair of CDH seemed to reverse pulmonary hypoplasia. However, these experiments did not recapitulate CDH because they were performed in the third trimester.

To mimic the human disease, the fetal lamb model of CDH was developed. Left-sided diaphragmatic hernias were created in fetal lambs at 60 days' gestation. The experimental group was repaired in the second trimester between 100 and 113 days' gestation before birth at term gestation,[25] whereas the control group was born at term gestation with a surgically created diaphragmatic hernia. Unrepaired fetal lambs had left lung hypoplasia, decreased number of pulmonary vessels per unit area of lung, and increased muscularization of the pulmonary arterial tree. However, surgical repair increased the lung volume and normalized pulmonary vascular density and medial wall thickness in the lung. These results were encouraging and became the basis for open fetal repair of CDH in human fetuses.

OPEN REPAIR IN HUMANS

Open fetal repair for CDH was developed because experiments in the fetal lamb model of CDH showed that in utero repair could salvage those with severe disease. Open fetal repair was attempted in 14 patients diagnosed before 24 weeks' gestation with severe left-sided CDH, mediastinal shift, and an intrathoracic stomach.[27] Only 4 patients survived. Even when repair of the diaphragmatic hernia was successful, pregnant mothers undergoing fetal surgery were plagued with problems such as preterm labor, uterine contractions, or uterine disruption. In addition, reducing the liver into the abdominal cavity compromised umbilical circulation through the umbilical vein and ductus venosus, leading to fetal demise. Open fetal repair of CDH was not technically feasible in patients with the worst prognosis.

To determine if open fetal repair was safe and efficacious for infants with liver-down CDH, a prospective trial was performed. Four fetuses underwent open fetal repair, whereas 7 fetuses underwent conventional postnatal repair.[28] There was no difference in survival: survival in the open fetal repair group was 75% and survival in patients undergoing standard postnatal diaphragmatic hernia repair was 86%. However, patients who underwent open fetal surgery did have a higher incidence of preterm delivery. The average gestational age of delivery was 32 weeks for patients undergoing open fetal repair, compared with 38 weeks for patients undergoing postnatal diaphragmatic hernia repair. Although open fetal surgery was technically feasible for patients with liver-down CDH, it did not offer a survival advantage over conventional postnatal care and also had a higher incidence of preterm birth.

Rationale for Tracheal Occlusion

The studies outlined earlier showed that pulmonary hypoplasia in diaphragmatic hernia was reversible and technically feasible in fetuses without liver herniation. However, open fetal repair did not show a survival benefit and therefore did not warrant the risk of possible preterm labor and infection. On the other hand, open fetal CDH repair was technically impossible in patients with liver herniation. As a result, alternative treatment options were explored. Tracheal occlusion originated from observations that patients with congenital high airway obstruction developed hyperplastic lungs. Pulmonary development is dependent on fetal breathing movements and a delicate balance between intraluminal pulmonary fluid and the surrounding amniotic fluid. The developing lung actively secretes fluid into the intra-alveolar space, and distension of the lung parenchyma is maintained with a closed glottis. Pulmonary hypoplasia can be induced by shunting amniotic fluid out of the uterus to produce oligohydramnios and by inhibiting fetal breathing with cervical cord transection.[29] In theory, tracheal occlusion would prevent the egress of intra-alveolar fluid and promote lung growth in utero.

Tracheal occlusion was studied extensively in the fetal lamb model of CDH. Various techniques to achieve tracheal occlusion were evaluated, including a foam-cuffed endotracheal tube, a foam plug,[30] and complete suture ligation.[31] Tracheal occlusion required a secure device that completely occluded the trachea without inadvertently damaging the trachea, and needed to be easily retrievable at birth to allow for respiration. Tracheal occlusion in fetal lambs with diaphragmatic hernias reduced herniated viscera into the abdomen and improved postnatal respiratory function.[30–32] Animals that underwent tracheal occlusion had increased lung volume, lung dry weight, lung DNA and protein, and alveolar surface area compared with animals without tracheal occlusion,[31–33] and these results were recapitulated with tracheal occlusion in the nitrofen rat model of CDH.[34] In addition, tracheal occlusion decreased pulmonary arteriolar medial wall thickness and muscularization in multiple animal models of CDH,[35–37] suggesting that tracheal occlusion can treat both pulmonary hypoplasia and pulmonary hypertension in CDH. However, tracheal occlusion decreased the number of type II pneumocytes and amount of surfactant expressed.[38–40] This effect was reversible with release of the occlusion device before birth.[38]

Tracheal Occlusion in Humans

Although open fetal repair of CDH was not technically feasible for fetuses with liver-up CDH, success in animal models with tracheal occlusion provided compelling evidence for fetal intervention. Therefore, tracheal occlusion was attempted using maternal laparotomy and open hysterotomy in 8 fetuses at the UCSF in 1996.[41] Various techniques were used to occlude the trachea, including an internal foam plug and external metal clips after fetal neck dissection. The optimal technique was to use 2 large opposing clips with a suture attached to each clip to facilitate removal at birth. Open fetal tracheal occlusion for CDH was a technique in evolution: complete occlusion often resulted in airway damage, like tracheomalacia or tracheal stenosis, whereas attempts to protect the fetal trachea resulted in incomplete occlusion and suboptimal lung growth.

Tracheal occlusion also posed a unique problem: it was an iatrogenic airway obstruction that would prevent gas exchange at birth. The occlusive device had to be removed and an airway had to be established while the fetus was still attached to placental circulation. A technique named the ex utero intrapartum treatment (EXIT) procedure was performed with the mother under general anesthesia.[42] A cesarean delivery was performed, the fetus was exteriorized, and a bronchoscope was used to monitor removal of the tracheal occlusion device. The trachea was repaired if necessary, and an airway was established with a tracheostomy or an endotracheal tube while fetal gas exchange was maintained through the placenta.

Between 1994 and 1997, 13 fetuses that were identified as having a poor prognosis (liver-up, and LHR <1.4) underwent open tracheal occlusion.[43] Survival was 15% in these 13 patients, but patients with a comparable severity who received standard postnatal therapy had a survival of 38%. In addition, the average gestational age at delivery for patients who underwent tracheal occlusion was 30 ± 0.6 weeks compared with 37.5 weeks ± 0.5 weeks for those who had standard postnatal repair. The low survival in the patients who underwent open tracheal occlusion was attributed to evolution of the open tracheal occlusion technique and preterm labor caused by a large uterine incision.

The Children's Hospital of Pennsylvania reported their experience with 15 cases of open fetal tracheal occlusion in patients with liver herniation and an LHR less than 1.0 in 2000.[44] The survival was 33% in patients undergoing tracheal occlusion, and causes of fetal and postnatal death were preterm birth, multisystem organ failure after prolonged intensive care and subsequent withdrawal of support, an atrial perforation from a central line, and inadequate lung growth. Although prenatal tracheal occlusion restored normal lung function in animal models, these 2 studies showed that hyperplastic lungs from tracheal occlusion were still functionally impaired in humans, and preterm birth was still an obstacle in fetal intervention.

Minimally Invasive Tracheal Occlusion

Despite advances in techniques with tracheal occlusion, preterm labor remained a problem because of the large uterine incision required for fetal exposure. In an effort to decrease problems with preterm labor, surgeons developed fetal endoscopic surgery (FETENDO), a technique that exposes the uterus through a maternal laparotomy and visualizes the fetus with a videoscopic camera through a small uterine incision. The FETENDO technique was applied to 8 fetuses with liver herniation and an LHR less than 1.4.[43] Performing FETENDO was a challenging technique because there was a mobile target (the fetus), variable placental location, tenuous membrane attachments, and a confined operating space. Initial attempts at FETENDO required conversion to an open procedure.

Nineteen patients with liver-up CDH and an LHR less than 1.4 underwent FETENDO temporary tracheal occlusion at UCSF.[23] The fetal trachea was dissected, a clip was placed on the trachea, and an EXIT procedure was used for delivery. Sixty-eight percent of patients survived. Twelve of 19 patients had separation of membranes and premature rupture of membranes. FETENDO did not seem to reduce maternal complications and a large retrospective study evaluating maternal morbidity after maternal-fetal surgery confirmed this finding: there were no differences in the incidence of premature rupture of membranes, placental abruption, or preterm delivery between endoscopic and open fetal surgery.[45] In addition, 7 of 13 patients who survived had complications related to tracheal dissection, such as vocal cord paralysis.

Complications with vocal cord paralysis using the FETENDO tracheal clip led to fetoscopic balloon tracheal occlusion to avoid damage to the recurrent laryngeal nerve from fetal neck dissection. Experiments in the fetal lamb model of CDH showed that fetoscopic tracheal occlusion using a detachable balloon successfully increased lung volume,[46,47] and eventually, temporary balloon tracheal occlusion was successfully completed in 2 fetuses through a single uterine port (**Fig. 1**).[48] Both of these patients had premature rupture of membranes approximately 1 month after the procedure

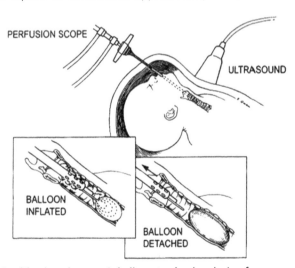

Fig. 1. Schematic of fetal tracheoscopic balloon tracheal occlusion for severe congenital diaphragmatic hernia. (*From* Harrison MR, Albanese CT, Hawgood SP, et al. Fetoscopic temporary tracheal occlusion by means of detachable balloon for congenital diaphragmatic hernia. Am J Obstet Gynecol 2001;185:732; with permission.)

and were delivered by EXIT procedure at 31 weeks' gestation. They required conventional ventilation for 1 week before postnatal repair of the diaphragmatic defect with a Gore-Tex patch reconstruction. Tracheomalacia was not observed in either patient, and both were discharged home at 37 and 39 weeks' gestation without oxygen.

RANDOMIZED CONTROLLED TRIAL FOR FETAL TRACHEAL OCCLUSION

Initial experience with fetal endoscopic balloon tracheal occlusion was encouraging, and a randomized controlled trial sponsored by the US National Institutes of Health was performed at UCSF to compare outcomes in prenatal tracheal occlusion against outcomes with standard postnatal care.[49] This study was performed in patients with a left-sided CDH, a normal echo and karyotype, with no other fetal anomalies, an LHR less than 1.4 measured between 22 and 28 weeks of gestation, and liver herniation. A maternal laparotomy was performed under general anesthesia. The first 2 patients underwent a 3-port fetal endoscopic tracheal clip. The protocol was revised after 2 patients underwent successful placement of a detachable tracheal balloon between the carina and vocal cords through a single 5-mm intrauterine port under ultrasound guidance. Fetuses were delivered by EXIT, during which the balloon tracheal occlusion device was deflated under direct visualization with bronchoscopy.

This trial was terminated early after 24 patients because there was a failure to detect a difference in survival at 90 days of life between the 11 patients who underwent fetoscopic tracheal occlusion and the 13 patients who received standard postnatal care. Survival for patients undergoing tracheal occlusion was 73%, whereas survival for patients who received standard postnatal care was 77%. The high survival in the control group was attributed to advances in postnatal care, such as gentle ventilation, high-frequency oscillatory ventilation, and permissive hypercapnea. There were no differences between the 2 groups in terms of the number of patients who needed ECMO, had chronic lung disease, hernia recurrence, gastroesophageal reflux disease, or failure to thrive. However, there was a significant increase in incidence of premature rupture of membranes: 100% of patients who had fetoscopic tracheal occlusion had premature rupture of membranes, whereas 23% of patients managed with standard postnatal care had premature rupture of membranes. Although fetoscopic balloon tracheal occlusion was technically feasible, this randomized controlled trial in the United States did not show a survival benefit over standard postnatal care.

TRACHEAL OCCLUSION: THE EUROPEAN EXPERIENCE

In Europe, significant advances have been made in tracheal occlusion for severe CDH. Procedures are performed completely percutaneously via a 3-mm fetoscope without need for a maternal laparotomy. A nonrandomized multicenter study was conducted on 210 fetuses with severe CDH to evaluate outcomes in patients who underwent fetal endoscopic tracheal occlusion (FETO).[50] The investigators reported that spontaneous preterm rupture of membranes occurred in 47% of patients and that FETO increased survival from 24% to 49% in left-sided CDH and from 0% to 35% in right-sided CDH. Both fetuses with either right-sided or left-sided CDH were included, and severity of CDH was based on o/e LHR. In contrast, the UCSF randomized controlled trial was limited to fetuses with left-sided CDH and an LHR less than 1.4. In addition, the European study was a nonrandomized study. In recent European experience, tracheal occlusion is reversed by removal of the tracheal balloon during a second fetoscopy before delivery. This strategy allows vaginal delivery when appropriate. In addition, reversal of tracheal occlusion may improve type II pneumocyte function and increase surfactant production. The results from the European experience are encouraging, and that approach is being studied in a prospective randomized controlled trial.

FUTURE DIRECTIONS FOR TRACHEAL OCCLUSION

Although prenatal complete balloon tracheal occlusion has been shown to cause lung hyperplasia in CDH, improved lung function has not been consistently shown in human trials. Complete tracheal occlusion interferes with dynamic pressure changes in the developing fetal lung that are associated with intrauterine fetal breathing. Dynamic tracheal occlusion devices are being developed that allow egress of intraluminal lung fluid through a pop-off valve.[51] These studies showed that oxygenation and lung compliance normalized in the lambs with CDH that underwent dynamic tracheal occlusion. These preliminary results suggest that to restore normal lung function and development, dynamic tracheal occlusion more realistically mimics normal fetal lung physiology than complete tracheal occlusion.

SUMMARY

More than 3 decades of research in multiple centers across the United States have led to significant advances in prenatal diagnosis, fetal treatment, and postnatal care of CDH. However, for those patients with severe disease, mortality still remains approximately 30%. Patients can now be stratified into low-risk and high-risk groups based on prenatal ultrasonography parameters, and expectant families can be counseled on treatment options and outcomes. Regardless, a solution has yet to be found for patients with severe CDH, and those with liver herniation and an LHR less than 1.0 remain at high risk for fetal demise, postnatal death, or long-term comorbidities, such as failure to thrive, oral aversion, and developmental delay. Multiple centers across the United States have established longitudinal outpatient clinics because infants with CDH are susceptible to long-term comorbidities. These longitudinal clinics can identify emerging problems, manage ongoing nutritional and developmental issues, and provide long-term follow-up to determine outcomes in CDH.

REFERENCES

1. Butler N, Claireaux AE. Congenital diaphragmatic hernia as a cause of perinatal mortality. Lancet 1962;1(7231):659–63.
2. de Buys Roessingh AS, Dinh-Xuan AT. Congenital diaphragmatic hernia: current status and review of the literature. Eur J Pediatr 2009;168(4):393–406.
3. Harrison MR. The unborn patient: the art and science of fetal therapy. 3rd edition. Philadelphia: WB Saunders; 2001.
4. Harrison MR, Adzick NS, Estes JM, et al. A prospective study of the outcome for fetuses with diaphragmatic hernia. JAMA 1994;271(5):382–4.
5. Harrison MR, Langer JC, Adzick NS, et al. Correction of congenital diaphragmatic hernia in utero, V. Initial clinical experience. J Pediatr Surg 1990;25(1): 47–55 [discussion: 56–7].
6. Adzick NS, Harrison MR, Glick PL, et al. Diaphragmatic hernia in the fetus: prenatal diagnosis and outcome in 94 cases. J Pediatr Surg 1985;20(4):357–61.
7. Heiss K, Manning P, Oldham KT, et al. Reversal of mortality for congenital diaphragmatic hernia with ECMO. Ann Surg 1989;209(2):225–30.
8. Metkus AP, Filly RA, Stringer MD, et al. Sonographic predictors of survival in fetal diaphragmatic hernia. J Pediatr Surg 1996;31(1):148–51 [discussion: 151–2].

9. Burge DM, Atwell JD, Freeman NV. Could the stomach site help predict outcome in babies with left sided congenital diaphragmatic hernia diagnosed antenatally? J Pediatr Surg 1989;24(6):567–9.

10. Hatch EI Jr, Kendall J, Blumhagen J. Stomach position as an in utero predictor of neonatal outcome in left-sided diaphragmatic hernia. J Pediatr Surg 1992;27(6): 778–9.

11. Crawford DC, Wright VM, Drake DP, et al. Fetal diaphragmatic hernia: the value of fetal echocardiography in the prediction of postnatal outcome. Br J Obstet Gynaecol 1989;96(6):705–10.

12. Albanese CT, Lopoo J, Goldstein RB, et al. Fetal liver position and perinatal outcome for congenital diaphragmatic hernia. Prenat Diagn 1998;18(11): 1138–42.

13. Kitano Y, Nakagawa S, Kuroda T, et al. Liver position in fetal congenital diaphragmatic hernia retains a prognostic value in the era of lung-protective strategy. J Pediatr Surg 2005;40(12):1827–32.

14. Jani J, Keller RL, Benachi A, et al. Prenatal prediction of survival in isolated left-sided diaphragmatic hernia. Ultrasound Obstet Gynecol 2006;27(1):18–22.

15. Arkovitz MS, Russo M, Devine P, et al. Fetal lung-head ratio is not related to outcome for antenatal diagnosed congenital diaphragmatic hernia. J Pediatr Surg 2007;42(1):107–10 [discussion: 110–1].

16. Peralta CF, Cavoretto P, Csapo B, et al. Assessment of lung area in normal fetuses at 12–32 weeks. Ultrasound in Obstetrics and Gynecology 2005;26(7): 718–24.

17. Jani J, Nicolaides KH, Keller RL, et al. Observed to expected lung area to head circumference ratio in the prediction of survival in fetuses with isolated diaphragmatic hernia. Ultrasound Obstet Gynecol 2007;30(1):67–71.

18. Deprest JA, Flemmer AW, Gratacos E, et al. Antenatal prediction of lung volume and in-utero treatment by fetal endoscopic tracheal occlusion in severe isolated congenital diaphragmatic hernia. Semin Fetal Neonatal Med 2009;14(1):8–13.

19. Paek BW, Coakley FV, Lu Y, et al. Congenital diaphragmatic hernia: prenatal evaluation with MR lung volumetry–preliminary experience. Radiology 2001;220(1): 63–7.

20. Lee TC, Lim FY, Keswani SG, et al. Late gestation fetal magnetic resonance imaging-derived total lung volume predicts postnatal survival and need for extracorporeal membrane oxygenation support in isolated congenital diaphragmatic hernia. J Pediatr Surg 2011;46(6):1165–71.

21. Worley KC, Dashe JS, Barber RG, et al. Fetal magnetic resonance imaging in isolated diaphragmatic hernia: volume of herniated liver and neonatal outcome. Am J Obstet Gynecol 2009;200(3):318, e1–6.

22. Kilian AK, Schaible T, Hofmann V, et al. Congenital diaphragmatic hernia: predictive value of MRI relative lung-to-head ratio compared with MRI fetal lung volume and sonographic lung-to-head ratio. AJR Am J Roentgenol 2009;192(1):153–8.

23. Harrison MR, Sydorak RM, Farrell JA, et al. Fetoscopic temporary tracheal occlusion for congenital diaphragmatic hernia: prelude to a randomized, controlled trial. J Pediatr Surg 2003;38(7):1012–20.

24. Harrison MR, Jester JA, Ross NA. Correction of congenital diaphragmatic hernia in utero. I. The model: intrathoracic balloon produces fatal pulmonary hypoplasia. Surgery 1980;88(1):174–82.

25. Adzick NS, Outwater KM, Harrison MR, et al. Correction of congenital diaphragmatic hernia in utero. IV. An early gestational fetal lamb model for pulmonary vascular morphometric analysis. J Pediatr Surg 1985;20(6):673–80.

26. Harrison MR, Bressack MA, Churg AM, et al. Correction of congenital diaphragmatic hernia in utero. II. Simulated correction permits fetal lung growth with survival at birth. Surgery 1980;88(2):260–8.
27. Harrison MR, Adzick NS, Flake AW, et al. Correction of congenital diaphragmatic hernia in utero: VI. Hard-earned lessons. J Pediatr Surg 1993;28(10):1411–7 [discussion: 1417–8].
28. Harrison MR, Adzick NS, Bullard KM, et al. Correction of congenital diaphragmatic hernia in utero VII: a prospective trial. J Pediatr Surg 1997;32(11): 1637–42.
29. Adzick NS, Harrison MR, Glick PL, et al. Experimental pulmonary hypoplasia and oligohydramnios: relative contributions of lung fluid and fetal breathing movements. J Pediatr Surg 1984;19(6):658–65.
30. Bealer JF, Skarsgard ED, Hedrick MH, et al. The 'PLUG' odyssey: adventures in experimental fetal tracheal occlusion. J Pediatr Surg 1995;30(2):361–4 [discussion: 364–5].
31. DiFiore JW, Fauza DO, Slavin R, et al. Experimental fetal tracheal ligation reverses the structural and physiological effects of pulmonary hypoplasia in congenital diaphragmatic hernia. J Pediatr Surg 1994;29(2):248–56 [discussion: 256–7].
32. Hedrick MH, Estes JM, Sullivan KM, et al. Plug the lung until it grows (PLUG): a new method to treat congenital diaphragmatic hernia in utero. J Pediatr Surg 1994;29(5):612–7.
33. Lipsett J, Cool JC, Runciman SI, et al. Effect of antenatal tracheal occlusion on lung development in the sheep model of congenital diaphragmatic hernia: a morphometric analysis of pulmonary structure and maturity. Pediatr Pulmonol 1998;25(4):257–69.
34. Kitano Y, Davies P, von Allmen D, et al. Fetal tracheal occlusion in the rat model of nitrofen-induced congenital diaphragmatic hernia. J Appl Physiol 1999;87(2): 769–75.
35. Kanai M, Kitano Y, von Allmen D, et al. Fetal tracheal occlusion in the rat model of nitrofen-induced congenital diaphragmatic hernia: tracheal occlusion reverses the arterial structural abnormality. J Pediatr Surg 2001;36(6):839–45.
36. Luks FI, Wild YK, Piasecki GJ, et al. Short-term tracheal occlusion corrects pulmonary vascular anomalies in the fetal lamb with diaphragmatic hernia. Surgery 2000;128(2):266–72.
37. Roubliova XI, Verbeken EK, Wu J, et al. Effect of tracheal occlusion on peripheric pulmonary vessel muscularization in a fetal rabbit model for congenital diaphragmatic hernia. Am J Obstet Gynecol 2004;191(3):830–6.
38. Bin Saddiq W, Piedboeuf B, Laberge JM, et al. The effects of tracheal occlusion and release on type II pneumocytes in fetal lambs. J Pediatr Surg 1997;32(6): 834–8.
39. Piedboeuf B, Laberge JM, Ghitulescu G, et al. Deleterious effect of tracheal obstruction on type II pneumocytes in fetal sheep. Pediatr Res 1997;41(4 Pt 1):473–9.
40. O'Toole SJ, Sharma A, Karamanoukian HL, et al. Tracheal ligation does not correct the surfactant deficiency associated with congenital diaphragmatic hernia. J Pediatr Surg 1996;31(4):546–50.
41. Harrison MR, Adzick NS, Flake AW, et al. Correction of congenital diaphragmatic hernia in utero VIII: response of the hypoplastic lung to tracheal occlusion. J Pediatr Surg 1996;31(10):339–48.
42. Mychaliska GB, Bealer JF, Graf JL, et al. Operating on placental support: the ex utero intrapartum treatment procedure. J Pediatr Surg 1997;32(2):227–30 [discussion: 230–1].

43. Harrison MR, Mychaliska GB, Albanese CT, et al. Correction of congenital diaphragmatic hernia in utero IX: fetuses with poor prognosis (liver herniation and low lung-to-head ratio) can be saved by fetoscopic temporary tracheal occlusion. J Pediatr Surg 1998;33(7):1017–22 [discussion: 1022–3].
44. Flake AW, Crombleholme TM, Johnson MP, et al. Treatment of severe congenital diaphragmatic hernia by fetal tracheal occlusion: clinical experience with fifteen cases. Am J Obstet Gynecol 2000;183(5):1059–66.
45. Golombeck K, Ball RH, Lee H, et al. Maternal morbidity after maternal-fetal surgery. Am J Obstet Gynecol 2006;194(3):834–9.
46. Deprest JA, Evrard VA, Van Ballaer PP, et al. Tracheoscopic endoluminal plugging using an inflatable device in the fetal lamb model. Eur J Obstet Gynecol Reprod Biol 1998;81(2):165–9.
47. Flageole H, Evrard VA, Vandenberghe K, et al. Tracheoscopic endotracheal occlusion in the ovine model: technique and pulmonary effects. J Pediatr Surg 1997;32(9):1328–31.
48. Harrison MR, Albanese CT, Hawgood SB, et al. Fetoscopic temporary tracheal occlusion by means of detachable balloon for congenital diaphragmatic hernia. Am J Obstet Gynecol 2001;185(3):730–3.
49. Harrison MR, Keller RL, Hawgood SB, et al. A randomized trial of fetal endoscopic tracheal occlusion for severe fetal congenital diaphragmatic hernia. N Engl J Med 2003;349(20):1916–24.
50. Jani JC, Nicolaides KH, Gratacos E, et al. Severe diaphragmatic hernia treated by fetal endoscopic tracheal occlusion. Ultrasound Obstet Gynecol 2009;34(3):304–10.
51. Jelin EB, Etemadi M, Encinas J, et al. Dynamic tracheal occlusion improves lung morphometrics and function in the fetal lamb model of congenital diaphragmatic hernia. J Pediatr Surg 2011;46(6):1150–7.

In Utero Hematopoietic Cell Transplantation for the Treatment of Congenital Anomalies

Amar Nijagal, MD[a], Alan W. Flake, MD[b], Tippi C. MacKenzie, MD[a],*

KEYWORDS

- In utero transplantation • Stem cell transplantation • Hematopoietic stem cells
- Engraftment • Chimerism • Maternal immune response

KEY POINTS

- In utero hematopoietic cell transplantation (IUHCTx) is a promising strategy for the treatment of common hematopoietic disorders and for inducing immune tolerance in the fetus.
- The delivery of cells into the early-gestation fetus offers the potential advantage of inducing donor-specific tolerance during the period of thymic education to self antigens.
- Animal models of IUHCTx have improved our understanding of the barriers limiting stem cell engraftment and have provided proof of concept for the treatment of several inherited disorders.
- The success of IUHCTx has not yet been realized in humans except in cases of immunodeficiencies.
- Recent studies have demonstrated that the maternal immune system plays a critical role in limiting engraftment in the fetus.

INTRODUCTION

Advances in our understanding of basic stem cell biology, prenatal diagnosis, and the technical aspects of fetal surgery have brought the use of in utero stem cell transplantation to treat congenital anomalies closer to clinical reality. Since its first description in 1982,[1] fetal intervention in patients has expanded to treat anatomic anomalies with both conventional and minimally invasive techniques.[2] The combination of high-resolution ultrasonography and prenatal molecular diagnostics has not only improved

[a] Eli and Edythe Broad Center of Regeneration Medicine and Stem Cell Research, Department of Surgery, 513 Parnassus Avenue, San Francisco, CA 94143-0570, USA; [b] Department of Surgery, The Children's Center for Fetal Research, The Children's Hospital of Philadelphia, University of Pennsylvania School of Medicine, 3615 Civic Center Boulevard, Philadelphia, PA 19104, USA
* Corresponding author.
E-mail address: tippi.mackenzie@ucsfmedctr.org

Clin Perinatol 39 (2012) 301–310
doi:10.1016/j.clp.2012.04.004
0095-5108/12/$ – see front matter © 2012 Elsevier Inc. All rights reserved.

the diagnosis of congenital conditions but has also provided a feasible way to deliver stem cells in the early-gestation fetus. Improved understanding of stem cell biology, prenatal diagnosis, and fetal surgical techniques has brought renewed interest and excitement for prenatal stem cell therapy.

The most promising applications of in utero stem cell therapy are for the treatment of common hematopoietic disorders such as sickle cell disease, thalassemias, and immunodeficiencies. The current standard treatment of these conditions involves bone marrow (BM) transplantation,[3–6] which is limited in its efficacy because of transplantation complications such as graft-versus-host disease (GVHD) or graft rejection, by the availability of few human leukocyte antigen (HLA)-matched donors, and by the morbidity of host myeloablation preceding transplantation.[6] The delivery of cells into the early-gestation fetus offers the potential advantage of inducing donor-specific tolerance, thus avoiding the toxicity of myeloablation and allowing for postnatal transplantation of allogeneic stem cells or organs.[7] The fetal environment can also promote the proliferation and differentiation of transplanted cells to facilitate widespread engraftment. Although the efficacy of in utero hematopoietic cell transplantation (IUHCTx) has been demonstrated in multiple small and large animal models, the clinical application of this technique in humans has had limited success. This article reviews the therapeutic rationale of IUHCTx, potential barriers to its applications, and recent experimental strategies to improve its clinical success.

THERAPEUTIC RATIONALE

The therapeutic rationale for IUHCTx is based on the numerous advantages that the fetal environment offers to allow for allogeneic (foreign) donor cell engraftment (reviewed in Ref.[7]). Specifically, the fetal environment may support the proliferation and migration of allogeneic donor cells. Hematopoietic stem cells (HSC) originate in the fetal yolk sac, migrate to the fetal liver, and eventually travel to the BM.[8,9] This relatively large-scale cellular migration could provide a favorable environment for donor cell homing and engraftment. Perhaps the most compelling reason to perform HSC transplantation in utero is the potential ability to achieve donor-specific tolerance. Theoretically, introducing allogeneic cells during the period of thymic education to self antigens should lead to deletion of allospecific T cells by negative selection.[10] The resulting antigen-specific tolerance that is established in utero can therefore minimize the need for myeloablation during postnatal cellular or organ transplantation.[11–13]

Experiments with nature have helped researchers understand the link between engraftment of foreign cells and antigen-specific tolerance. Dizygotic cattle share placental circulation and have secondary long-term engraftment of foreign cells from their siblings, resulting in donor-specific tolerance.[14] Similar observations have been made in human twins, for whom chimerism has led to a lack of alloreactivity between the two siblings.[15] Examples of natural chimerism in other animals have also been reported,[16,17] with levels of engraftment high enough to be potentially therapeutic for hematologic diseases.[7] An important caveat to these findings is that the constant antigen exposure that begins early in gestation in nature poses challenges when attempting to reproduce this process using animal models of IUHCTx, in which transplantation of allogeneic donor cells is performed during mid-gestation (reviewed in Ref.[7]). Nevertheless, these observations support the concept that hematopoietic chimerism established in utero induces immune tolerance.

The idea of using the fetal environment to induce tolerance is supported by the rich literature on tolerance to noninherited maternal antigens (NIMAs). The natural trafficking of maternal cells into the fetus (maternal microchimerism) leads to the generation of regulatory T cells that prevent an antimaternal immune response by the fetus.[18] Although the levels of maternal cells in the fetus are low, the presence of microchimerism may have implications for the success of postnatal transplantation when maternal cells are used. For example, the authors recently showed that patients with biliary atresia, in whom there is a higher level of baseline maternal microchimerism,[19] have less graft failure when they receive a liver from their mother.[20] In the setting of kidney transplantation, improved graft survival has been observed if the haplotype mismatched sibling expresses NIMAs compared with donors that express noninherited paternal antigens, demonstrating the tolerogenic effect of NIMAs.[21] NIMA exposure also has a beneficial effect on outcomes after BM transplantation.[22] These observations support the idea that tolerance may be induced even with low levels of engraftment and that a viable treatment strategy for congenital stem cell disorders is to induce tolerance in utero, followed by postnatal booster transplants to achieve therapeutic levels of donor cells.[11,23,24]

ANIMAL EXPERIENCE WITH IUHCTx

The use of animal models of IUHCTx has greatly improved our understanding of the barriers involved with successful stem cell engraftment and has provided proof of concept for the treatment of several inherited disorders (**Table 1**). The earliest experience with IUHCTx comes from the seminal experiments of Billingham and colleagues[25] in which in utero transplantation of allogeneic cells led to donor-specific tolerance to skin grafts in mice. It was soon noted that immunodeficient mice engraft more efficiently, likely secondary to a competitive advantage of the transplanted cells in such an environment.[26–29]

Early studies of IUHCTx using immunocompetent, wild-type recipient mice were limited by poor rates of engraftment. More recently, modifications to the IUHCTx technique have allowed for the delivery of higher cell numbers, resulting in macroscopic levels of donor cells that are detectable by flow cytometry.[30] Since the technical barriers to achieving high levels of engraftment in mice have been largely overcome, current research using this model has focused on the mechanisms by which donor-specific tolerance is achieved. In a mixed lymphocyte reaction, the authors have demonstrated that there are fewer allospecific host T cells in chimeras than in normal controls, suggesting that clonal deletion is an important mechanism in the establishment of chimerism.[31,32] Previous work has also implicated anergy as a tolerance mechanism after

Table 1
Successful treatment of inherited disorders using animal models of IUHCTx

Disease	Animal Model	Defective Gene	References
Anemia	Mouse	c-kit tyrosine kinase	27,28,66
Autosomal recessive osteoporosis	Mouse	Tcirg1	67,68
Leukocyte adhesion deficiency	Dog	Leukocyte integrin CD18	24
Osteogenesis imperfecta	Mouse	Col1a1	69
Severe combined immunodeficiency	Mouse	Scid	26,61,70–72
Sickle cell disease	Mouse	α-Globin	23
Thalassemia	Mouse	β-Globin	23

IUHCTx.[33] Recent data suggest that induction of donor-specific Tregs may also be a critical mechanism of tolerance (Nijagal A and MacKenzie TC, unpublished observations, 2012).[31,34] Remarkably, stable engraftment of even low levels of allogeneic HSC (<1%–2% engraftment) in mice has uniformly led to postnatal tolerance to the donor antigen. These data support the notion that tolerance depends on achieving a threshold level of engraftment[35] and on maintaining chimerism in the host.

Experience in large animal models has also shown multilineage engraftment of donor cells, providing support for the biology and technical feasibility of in utero transplantation. The sheep model was the first large animal model to demonstrate engraftment of allogeneic cells after fetal transplantation.[36] Sheep have been a particularly useful tool for the study of engraftment of human cells, because the xenogeneic cells are not rejected, they can be tracked easily, and their levels can be boosted using human granulocyte-colony stimulating factor.[37–39] IUHCTx in sheep provides a natural, unperturbed environment in which to study the engraftment and differentiation capacity of human stem cells such as embryonic[40] and mesenchymal stem cells.[41] Similar to sheep, the canine model readily accepts xenogeneic transplants.[42] Multilineage engraftment has been demonstrated in hematologically normal dogs,[24] and IUHCTx with postnatal boosting has successfully cured the canine equivalent of human leukocyte adhesion deficiency.[24] Using the pig model of IUHCTx, induction of immune tolerance in the fetus has proved to be beneficial for postnatal solid organ transplantation. IUHCTx (using adult BM-derived HSC) in fetal swine led to prolonged survival of a kidney allograft,[43] providing experimental support for the use of this strategy in fetuses with congenital anomalies requiring postnatal organ transplantation. Finally, low levels of engraftment have been seen in nonhuman primates.[44–46] Although the human immune system will present its own unique challenges, these large animal models demonstrate the technical feasibility of in utero transplantation and confirm the potential to achieve stable engraftment after IUHCTx in an immunocompetent host.

HUMAN CLINICAL EXPERIENCE

The success of IUHCTx in large animal models has not yet been realized in humans except in cases of immunodeficiencies (reviewed in Ref.[47]). The first transplantation was performed in a fetus with bare lymphocyte syndrome.[48] Subsequent to this report, several studies described the successful treatment of severe combined immunodeficiency (SCID) with IUHCTx.[49–53] In these cases either fetal liver, paternal BM, or maternal BM-derived CD34+ cells were transplanted between 16 and 26 weeks' gestation, and resulted in engraftment of donor cells at birth. Follow-up at 4 years was reported for one of these patients,[47] who continued to have cellular reconstitution and intact immune responses to vaccinations. This patient remains healthy, without clinically significant infections at 15 years of age (Flake AW, unpublished observation, 2012).

Attempts at using IUHCTx to treat diseases other than SCID have been unsuccessful, and have led investigators to study the barriers that limit transplantation success (reviewed in Ref.[47]). Identifying common factors that lead to poor engraftment is challenging, as there are many variables among these reported cases. For example, transplantations occurred at different centers, donor cells were obtained from different sources, and the transplantations were performed at varying gestational ages. The inherent variability in these studies has made it difficult to attribute the lack of success to any one specific factor, necessitating the use of animal models to gain insight into the barriers that limit engraftment after IUHCTx.

FACTORS LIMITING ENGRAFTMENT AFTER IUHCTx

Poor engraftment after IUHCTx is due to several factors.[47] Donor cells could be at a competitive disadvantage when transplanted into an intact fetal host. Alternatively, a limited number of hematopoietic niches could exist for donor cells. There is also evidence to suggest that the allogeneic cells transplanted in utero are susceptible to rejection by an immune response. Animal models have been used to study the contribution of each of these factors to donor cell engraftment.

The idea that donor cells may have a competitive disadvantage in the fetal environment is supported by observations in adult animals that conferring a survival advantage to donor cells leads to higher rates of engraftment. When using c-kit knockout mice with a deficiency of host HSC proliferation, for example, full immune reconstitution is demonstrated after the transplantation of only 1 or 2 donor HSC.[54] Furthermore, engraftment after postnatal BM transplantation is maintained consistently despite a relatively lower number of transplanted cells in an irradiated host where host competition is eliminated.[55] Modifications to the host hematopoietic environment that maintain SDF1-α induced migration[56] or inhibit fetal hematopoiesis[57] may improve donor-cell homing and engraftment, but clinical applications will need significant testing to ensure safety.

The number of available niches and the proliferative capacity of the fetal environment add to the competitive disadvantage of donor allografts. In adult mice, selective depletion of host HSC before BM transplant results in high rates of engraftment, suggesting that vacating host stem cell niches may improve chimerism after IUHCTx.[58] The possibility that there is a finite number of available hematopoietic niches for donor cell engraftment is supported by the observation that increasing the dose of donor cells results in an eventual plateau of engraftment efficiency in an allogeneic and xenogeneic fetal lamb model.[59] Studies have also demonstrated that the proliferative nature of the fetal environment contributes to the host's competitive advantage. Donor BM cells rapidly home to the fetal liver after IUHCTx, followed by a decrease of donor cell engraftment, demonstrating the ability of host cells to outcompete donor HSC.[60] Intrinsic proliferative properties of fetal liver cells likely accounts for the advantage of the host, thus providing an explanation for the poor engraftment seen when adult BM cells are transplanted in humans.[61] Despite these obstacles, the mouse model of IUHCTx has demonstrated that transplantation of large numbers of donor cells can result in multilineage engraftment.

The host (fetal) immune response has been thought to be the main barrier to donor cell engraftment; however, recent studies have demonstrated that the maternal immune system in fact plays a critical role in limiting engraftment in the fetus. The authors have demonstrated that when adult allogeneic cells are used for IUHCTx a maternal immune response is induced, and maternal antibodies transmitted in breast milk cause an adaptive alloimmune response in the pups, resulting in donor cell loss.[31] In a separate study using fetal liver–derived donor cells, the authors have shown that maternal T cells are critical for the engraftment of allogeneic donor cells in mice. Matching donor cells to the mother in immunocompetent mice led to a significant improvement in the rates of engraftment with allogeneic donor cells.[32] These data demonstrate that the maternal immune response is likely the predominant factor that determines whether successful engraftment can occur. Improved understanding of the fetal immune response may still, however, reveal host factors that are important for engraftment. For example, a threshold of chimerism is likely required to allow for effective antigen presentation in the thymus and periphery, both of which are required for the induction of tolerance mechanisms.[35]

COMPLICATIONS

Compared with more invasive open fetal surgery procedures, fetal stem cell transplantation is technically simpler and is generally well tolerated. The minimally invasive nature of in utero cellular transplantation decreases the chances for preterm labor or membrane separation, both of which are common after more invasive fetal procedures.[62] Whereas GVHD is a common complication after postnatal BM transplantation,[6] it is rarely observed even when mature T cells are transplanted in utero. There has been only one reported case in humans with GVHD after IUHCTx. In this case, a fetus died at 20 weeks' gestation after receiving CD34-enriched BM cells, and at autopsy was found to have overwhelming myelopoiesis. Achieving an optimum level of T-cell depletion can lead to successful engraftment and mitigate the small risk of GVHD after IUHCTx.[43]

FUTURE DIRECTIONS

IUHCTx holds great promise for the treatment of congenital hematopoietic diseases. The ability to induce immune tolerance using this technique allows for postnatal booster transplants to enhance engraftment without the need for postnatal myeloablation. As the understanding of stem cell differentiation continues to improve, the therapeutic applications of in utero transplantation should expand to include the treatment of nonhematopoietic stem cell disorders such as muscular dystrophy[63] or single-gene disorders such as hemophilia.[64] It is also possible that in the era of personalized medicine, genetically modified patient-matched induced pluripotent stem cells can be grown from samples of placental chorionic villus.[65] Given the financial constraints to generating patient-specific HSC, tissue banks containing HLA-matched embryonic stem cells can be used as a source of HSC for transplantation. However, any clinical application of such strategies must overcome the current bottleneck in the differentiation of these cells along the hematopoietic lineage in vivo. Advances in generating patient-specific and disease-specific HSC should also take into account the need for matching major histocompatibility complex on donor cells to the mother, to decrease the chances of rejection by the maternal immune system.

IUHCTx is at a critical junction. Not only have the barriers that once limited its success been overcome, but improved understanding of stem cell biology has provided a potentially rich and diverse source of donor cells. These factors have reinvigorated the field and have expanded the potential of this treatment strategy for new clinical applications.

REFERENCES

1. Harrison MR, Golbus MS, Filly RA, et al. Fetal surgery for congenital hydronephrosis. N Engl J Med 1982;306(10):591–3.
2. Sydorak RM, Nijagal A, Albanese CT. Endoscopic techniques in fetal surgery. Yonsei Med J 2001;42(6):695–710.
3. Johnson FL, Look AT, Gockerman J, et al. Bone-marrow transplantation in a patient with sickle-cell anemia. N Engl J Med 1984;311(12):780–3.
4. Kamani N, August CS, Douglas SD, et al. Bone marrow transplantation in chronic granulomatous disease. J Pediatr 1984;105(1):42–6.
5. Lucarelli G, Galimberti M, Polchi P, et al. Bone marrow transplantation in patients with thalassemia. N Engl J Med 1990;322(7):417–21.
6. Parkman R. The application of bone marrow transplantation to the treatment of genetic diseases. Science 1986;232(4756):1373–8.

7. Santore MT, Roybal JL, Flake AW. Prenatal stem cell transplantation and gene therapy. Clin Perinatol 2009;36(2):451–71, xi.
8. Elder M, Golbus MS, Cowan MJ. Ontogeny of T- and B-cell immunity. In: Edwards RG, editor. Fetal tissue transplants in medicine. Cambridge (UK): University Press; 1992. p. 97–128.
9. Medvinsky A, Dzierzak E. Definitive hematopoiesis is autonomously initiated by the AGM region. Cell 1996;86(6):897–906.
10. Palmer E. Negative selection—clearing out the bad apples from the T-cell repertoire. Nat Rev Immunol 2003;3(5):383–91.
11. Ashizuka S, Peranteau WH, Hayashi S, et al. Busulfan-conditioned bone marrow transplantation results in high-level allogeneic chimerism in mice made tolerant by in utero hematopoietic cell transplantation. Exp Hematol 2006;34(3):359–68.
12. Hayashi S, Peranteau WH, Shaaban AF, et al. Complete allogeneic hematopoietic chimerism achieved by a combined strategy of in utero hematopoietic stem cell transplantation and postnatal donor lymphocyte infusion. Blood 2002;100(3):804–12.
13. Peranteau WH, Hayashi S, Hsieh M, et al. High-level allogeneic chimerism achieved by prenatal tolerance induction and postnatal nonmyeloablative bone marrow transplantation. Blood 2002;100(6):2225–34.
14. Owen RD. Immunogenetic consequences of vascular anastomoses between bovine twins. Science 1945;102(2651):400–1.
15. Thomsen M, Hansen HE, Dickmeiss E. MLC and CML studies in the family of a pair of HLA haploidentical chimeric twins. Scand J Immunol 1977;6(5):523–8.
16. Picus J, Aldrich WR, Letvin NL. A naturally occurring bone-marrow-chimeric primate. I. Integrity of its immune system. Transplantation 1985;39(3):297–303.
17. Picus J, Holley K, Aldrich WR, et al. A naturally occurring bone marrow-chimeric primate. II. Environment dictates restriction on cytolytic T lymphocyte-target cell interactions. J Exp Med 1985;162(6):2035–52.
18. Mold JE, Michaelsson J, Burt TD, et al. Maternal alloantigens promote the development of tolerogenic fetal regulatory T cells in utero. Science 2008;322(5907):1562–5.
19. Suskind DL, Rosenthal P, Heyman MB, et al. Maternal microchimerism in the livers of patients with biliary atresia. BMC Gastroenterol 2004;4:14.
20. Nijagal A, Fleck S, Hills NK, et al. Decreased risk of graft failure with maternal liver transplantation in patients with biliary atresia. Am J Transplant 2012;12(2):409–19.
21. Burlingham WJ, Grailer AP, Heisey DM, et al. The effect of tolerance to noninherited maternal HLA antigens on the survival of renal transplants from sibling donors. N Engl J Med 1998;339(23):1657–64.
22. van Rood JJ, Loberiza FR Jr, Zhang MJ, et al. Effect of tolerance to noninherited maternal antigens on the occurrence of graft-versus-host disease after bone marrow transplantation from a parent or an HLA-haploidentical sibling. Blood 2002;99(5):1572–7.
23. Hayashi S, Abdulmalik O, Peranteau WH, et al. Mixed chimerism following in utero hematopoietic stem cell transplantation in murine models of hemoglobinopathy. Exp Hematol 2003;31(2):176–84.
24. Peranteau WH, Heaton TE, Gu YC, et al. Haploidentical in utero hematopoietic cell transplantation improves phenotype and can induce tolerance for postnatal same-donor transplants in the canine leukocyte adhesion deficiency model. Biol Blood Marrow Transplant 2009;15(3):293–305.
25. Billingham RE, Brent L, Medawar PB. Actively acquired tolerance of foreign cells. Nature 1953;172(4379):603–6.

26. Blazar BR, Taylor PA, Vallera DA. In utero transfer of adult bone marrow cells into recipients with severe combined immunodeficiency disorder yields lymphoid progeny with T- and B-cell functional capabilities. Blood 1995;86(11):4353–66.

27. Blazar BR, Taylor PA, Vallera DA. Adult bone marrow-derived pluripotent hematopoietic stem cells are engraftable when transferred in utero into moderately anemic fetal recipients. Blood 1995;85(3):833–41.

28. Fleischman RA, Mintz B. Prevention of genetic anemias in mice by microinjection of normal hematopoietic stem cells into the fetal placenta. Proc Natl Acad Sci U S A 1979;76(11):5736–40.

29. Fleischman RA, Mintz B. Development of adult bone marrow stem cells in H-2-compatible and -incompatible mouse fetuses. J Exp Med 1984;159(3): 731–45.

30. Peranteau WH, Endo M, Adibe OO, et al. Evidence for an immune barrier after in utero hematopoietic-cell transplantation. Blood 2007;109(3):1331–3.

31. Merianos DJ, Tiblad E, Santore MT, et al. Maternal alloantibodies induce a postnatal immune response that limits engraftment following in utero hematopoietic cell transplantation in mice. J Clin Invest 2009;119(9):2590–600.

32. Nijagal A, Wegorzewska M, Jarvis E, et al. Maternal T cells limit engraftment after in utero hematopoietic cell transplantation in mice. J Clin Invest 2011;121(2): 582–92.

33. Kim HB, Shaaban AF, Milner R, et al. In utero bone marrow transplantation induces donor-specific tolerance by a combination of clonal deletion and clonal anergy. J Pediatr Surg 1999;34(5):726–9 [discussion: 9–30].

34. Hayashi S, Hsieh M, Peranteau WH, et al. Complete allogeneic hematopoietic chimerism achieved by in utero hematopoietic cell transplantation and cotransplantation of LLME-treated, MHC-sensitized donor lymphocytes. Exp Hematol 2004;32(3):290–9.

35. Durkin ET, Jones KA, Rajesh D, et al. Early chimerism threshold predicts sustained engraftment and NK-cell tolerance in prenatal allogeneic chimeras. Blood 2008;112(13):5245–53.

36. Flake AW, Harrison MR, Adzick NS, et al. Transplantation of fetal hematopoietic stem cells in utero: the creation of hematopoietic chimeras. Science 1986; 233(4765):776–8.

37. Almeida-Porada G, Porada C, Gupta N, et al. The human-sheep chimeras as a model for human stem cell mobilization and evaluation of hematopoietic grafts' potential. Exp Hematol 2007;35(10):1594–600.

38. Zanjani ED, Flake AW, Rice H, et al. Long-term repopulating ability of xenogeneic transplanted human fetal liver hematopoietic stem cells in sheep. J Clin Invest 1994;93(3):1051–5.

39. Zanjani ED, Pallavicini MG, Ascensao JL, et al. Engraftment and long-term expression of human fetal hemopoietic stem cells in sheep following transplantation in utero. J Clin Invest 1992;89(4):1178–88.

40. Narayan AD, Chase JL, Lewis RL, et al. Human embryonic stem cell-derived hematopoietic cells are capable of engrafting primary as well as secondary fetal sheep recipients. Blood 2006;107(5):2180–3.

41. Liechty KW, MacKenzie TC, Shaaban AF, et al. Human mesenchymal stem cells engraft and demonstrate site-specific differentiation after in utero transplantation in sheep. Nat Med 2000;6(11):1282–6.

42. Omori F, Lutzko C, Abrams-Ogg A, et al. Adoptive transfer of genetically modified human hematopoietic stem cells into preimmune canine fetuses. Exp Hematol 1999;27(2):242–9.

43. Lee PW, Cina RA, Randolph MA, et al. In utero bone marrow transplantation induces kidney allograft tolerance across a full major histocompatibility complex barrier in swine. Transplantation 2005;79(9):1084–90.
44. Shields LE, Gaur LK, Gough M, et al. In utero hematopoietic stem cell transplantation in nonhuman primates: the role of T cells. Stem Cells 2003;21(3):304–14.
45. Tarantal AF, Goldstein O, Barley F, et al. Transplantation of human peripheral blood stem cells into fetal rhesus monkeys (*Macaca mulatta*). Transplantation 2000;69(9):1818–23.
46. Asano T, Ageyama N, Takeuchi K, et al. Engraftment and tumor formation after allogeneic in utero transplantation of primate embryonic stem cells. Transplantation 2003;76(7):1061–7.
47. Flake AW, Zanjani ED. In utero hematopoietic stem cell transplantation: ontogenic opportunities and biologic barriers. Blood 1999;94(7):2179–91.
48. Touraine JL, Raudrant D, Royo C, et al. In-utero transplantation of stem cells in bare lymphocyte syndrome. Lancet 1989;1(8651):1382.
49. Flake AW, Roncarolo MG, Puck JM, et al. Treatment of X-linked severe combined immunodeficiency by in utero transplantation of paternal bone marrow. N Engl J Med 1996;335(24):1806–10.
50. Wengler GS, Lanfranchi A, Frusca T, et al. In-utero transplantation of parental CD34 haematopoietic progenitor cells in a patient with X-linked severe combined immunodeficiency (SCIDXI). Lancet 1996;348(9040):1484–7.
51. Touraine JL, Raudrant D, Laplace S. Transplantation of hemopoietic cells from the fetal liver to treat patients with congenital diseases postnatally or prenatally. Transplant Proc 1997;29(1-2):712–3.
52. Gil J, Porta F, Bartolome J, et al. Immune reconstitution after in utero bone marrow transplantation in a fetus with severe combined immunodeficiency with natural killer cells. Transplant Proc 1999;31(6):2581.
53. Pirovano S, Notarangelo LD, Malacarne F, et al. Reconstitution of T-cell compartment after in utero stem cell transplantation: analysis of T-cell repertoire and thymic output. Haematologica 2004;89(4):450–61.
54. Mintz B, Anthony K, Litwin S. Monoclonal derivation of mouse myeloid and lymphoid lineages from totipotent hematopoietic stem cells experimentally engrafted in fetal hosts. Proc Natl Acad Sci U S A 1984;81(24):7835–9.
55. Stewart FM, Zhong S, Wuu J, et al. Lymphohematopoietic engraftment in minimally myeloablated hosts. Blood 1998;91(10):3681–7.
56. Peranteau WH, Endo M, Adibe OO, et al. CD26 inhibition enhances allogeneic donor-cell homing and engraftment after in utero hematopoietic-cell transplantation. Blood 2006;108(13):4268–74.
57. Lindton B, Tolfvenstam T, Norbeck O, et al. Recombinant parvovirus B19 empty capsids inhibit fetal hematopoietic colony formation in vitro. Fetal Diagn Ther 2001;16(1):26–31.
58. Czechowicz A, Kraft D, Weissman IL, et al. Efficient transplantation via antibody-based clearance of hematopoietic stem cell niches. Science 2007;318(5854):1296–9.
59. Flake AW, Zanjani ED. Cellular therapy. Obstet Gynecol Clin North Am 1997; 24(1):159–77.
60. Shaaban AF, Kim HB, Milner R, et al. A kinetic model for the homing and migration of prenatally transplanted marrow. Blood 1999;94(9):3251–7.
61. Taylor PA, McElmurry RT, Lees CJ, et al. Allogenic fetal liver cells have a distinct competitive engraftment advantage over adult bone marrow cells when infused into fetal as compared with adult severe combined immunodeficient recipients. Blood 2002;99(5):1870–2.

62. Golombeck K, Ball RH, Lee H, et al. Maternal morbidity after maternal-fetal surgery. Am J Obstet Gynecol 2006;194(3):834–9.
63. Mackenzie TC, Shaaban AF, Radu A, et al. Engraftment of bone marrow and fetal liver cells after in utero transplantation in MDX mice. J Pediatr Surg 2002;37(7): 1058–64.
64. Sabatino DE, Mackenzie TC, Peranteau W, et al. Persistent expression of hF.IX After tolerance induction by in utero or neonatal administration of AAV-1-F.IX in hemophilia B mice. Mol Ther 2007;15(9):1677–85.
65. Ye L, Chang JC, Lin C, et al. Induced pluripotent stem cells offer new approach to therapy in thalassemia and sickle cell anemia and option in prenatal diagnosis in genetic diseases. Proc Natl Acad Sci U S A 2009;106(24):9826–30.
66. Howson-Jan K, Matloub YH, Vallera DA, et al. In utero engraftment of fully H-2-incompatible versus congenic adult bone marrow transferred into nonanemic or anemic murine fetal recipients. Transplantation 1993;56(3):709–16.
67. Frattini A, Blair HC, Sacco MG, et al. Rescue of ATPa3-deficient murine malignant osteopetrosis by hematopoietic stem cell transplantation in utero. Proc Natl Acad Sci U S A 2005;102(41):14629–34.
68. Tondelli B, Blair HC, Guerrini M, et al. Fetal liver cells transplanted in utero rescue the osteopetrotic phenotype in the oc/oc mouse. Am J Pathol 2009;174(3): 727–35.
69. Panaroni C, Gioia R, Lupi A, et al. In utero transplantation of adult bone marrow decreases perinatal lethality and rescues the bone phenotype in the knockin murine model for classical, dominant osteogenesis imperfecta. Blood 2009; 114(2):459–68.
70. Archer DR, Turner CW, Yeager AM, et al. Sustained multilineage engraftment of allogeneic hematopoietic stem cells in NOD/SCID mice after in utero transplantation. Blood 1997;90(8):3222–9.
71. Liuba K, Pronk CJ, Stott SR, et al. Polyclonal T-cell reconstitution of X-SCID recipients after in utero transplantation of lymphoid-primed multipotent progenitors. Blood 2009;113(19):4790–8.
72. Waldschmidt TJ, Panoskaltsis-Mortari A, McElmurry RT, et al. Abnormal T cell-dependent B-cell responses in SCID mice receiving allogeneic bone marrow in utero. Severe combined immune deficiency. Blood 2002;100(13):4557–64.

Advances in Neonatal Extracorporeal Support

The Role of Extracorporeal Membrane Oxygenation and the Artificial Placenta

Brian W. Gray, MD[a], Andrew W. Shaffer, MD, MS[a,c],
George B. Mychaliska, MD[b,*]

KEYWORDS

- Extracorporeal membrane oxygenation • ECMO • Extracorporeal life support
- Neonatal • Respiratory failure • Cardiac failure • Artificial placenta • EXIT to ECMO
- Prematurity

KEY POINTS

- Extracorporeal membrane oxygenation (ECMO) is currently indicated for neonates 34 weeks or more estimated gestational age weighing 2.0 kg or more; however, evidence suggests that smaller and more premature infants may benefit.
- Use of ECMO peaked in 1992 and has declined since that time, primarily because of improvements in other forms of critical care life support. To some extent, these improvements have been realized as a result of lessons learned from the early ECMO experience.
- Ex utero intrapartum therapy to ECMO may be used in late-term fetuses with anticipated respiratory and/or cardiac failure at birth, but the indications and efficacy remain unproven.
- The artificial placenta is theoretically an ideal extracorporeal support strategy for extremely premature infants because it recapitulates the intrauterine environment and maintains fetal circulation without mechanical ventilation.
- Animal studies using an umbilical arteriovenous artificial placenta have met with limited success in the past. Contemporary studies support a venovenous mode of support, which obviates many inherent problems with arteriovenous strategy.
- Many challenges remain in the development of the artificial placenta before clinical translation.

[a] Section of Pediatric Surgery, C.S. Mott Children's Hospital, University of Michigan Health System, B560 MSRBII, 1150 West Medical Center Drive, Ann Arbor, MI 48109, USA; [b] Section of Pediatric Surgery, Fetal Diagnosis and Treatment Center, C.S. Mott Children's Hospital, University of Michigan Health System, 1540 East Hospital Drive, SPC 4211, Ann Arbor, MI 48109, USA; [c] Department of General Surgery, William Beaumont Health System, 3601 West 13 Mile Road, Royal Oak, Detroit, MI 48073, USA
* Corresponding author.
E-mail address: mychalis@med.umich.edu

Clin Perinatol 39 (2012) 311–329
doi:10.1016/j.clp.2012.04.006
0095-5108/12/$ – see front matter © 2012 Elsevier Inc. All rights reserved.

perinatology.theclinics.com

PROGRESS IN PERINATAL/NEONATAL EXTRACORPOREAL MEMBRANE OXYGENATION
Neonatal Extracorporeal Membrane Oxygenation: Past, Present, and Future

Robert Bartlett and his group had been studying extracorporeal support in laboratory animals for 10 years before the first neonatal extracorporeal membrane oxygenation (ECMO) patient was supported in 1975; this clinical application signified a radical shift in the treatment paradigm for neonatal respiratory failure.[1] The neonate, Esperanza, was suffering from respiratory failure secondary to meconium aspiration that was recalcitrant to conventional ventilator support. She was successfully supported and now is 37 years old.[2]

The currently accepted treatment of perinatal/neonatal cardiopulmonary failure includes low-volume protective ventilation,[3] inhaled nitric oxide,[4,5] surfactant therapy,[6,7] and high-frequency oscillatory ventilation.[8] If the cardiac or pulmonary failure is refractory to maximal medical therapy then ECMO should be considered.[9,10] The standard application of ECMO is primarily limited to neonates 34 weeks or more estimated gestational age (EGA) and weighing 2 kg or more. Clinical experience and laboratory work suggest extracorporeal support may be effective at lower gestational ages by using Preemie ECMO or the artificial placenta (**Table 1**).

History of Extracorporeal Life Support

John Gibbon is credited with envisioning total cardiopulmonary support in 1939. He published the first successful heart surgery with assistance of the heart-lung machine in 1954.[11] Lillehei and his group in Minnesota were the first to perform extracorporeal support of pediatric patients. In 1955, they published a series of 8 pediatric cardiac patients using the parents as the support mechanism.[12] This opened the door for the first successful application of ECMO in the clinical setting by J. Donald Hill in 1971.[13] The application of ECMO for postoperative cardiopulmonary failure in children was described as early as 1972.[14] The first series of neonatal patients was published in 1982, and reported 45 cases with a survival rate of 50%.[15] The first prospective randomized trials of ECMO for neonatal respiratory failure were published in 1985 and 1989. These 2 studies demonstrated high rates of survival (100% and 94%, respectively) in neonatal patients with respiratory failure. The first trial was published by the group at Michigan, and was criticized for both exposing neonates to the risks of ECMO and for having too few patients in the control arm.[16] Ironically, 2 years later the Boston trial was criticized for denying ECMO to too many patients in the control limb of the study.[17] Despite early criticism and skepticism of this novel treatment, by 1986 there were 18 centers with successful neonatal ECMO teams.[18] The early ECMO community was a model of professional collaboration. The Extracorporeal Life Support Organization (ELSO) was founded in 1989 and maintained a registry of extracorporeal life support (ECLS) cases, developed standard guidelines and practices, and published the textbook on ECLS known as the

Table 1 ECLS modality by age group																
Gestational age (wk)	24	25	26	27	28	29	30	31	32	33	34	35	36	37	38	39	40
ECLS treatment modality	Artificial placenta[a]					Preemie ECMO[b]					ECMO[c]						

[a] Laboratory research.
[b] Clinically feasible.
[c] Standard of care.

Red Book.[19] The ELSO database has provided data for 2 additional prospective trials of ECMO in newborns as well as numerous other clinical studies.[20,21] These trials provided substantive evidence that ECMO was beneficial in neonatal patients with respiratory failure. As ECMO treatment evolved beyond cardiopulmonary support, the term ECLS has emerged to encompass all of the assistive therapies available, including cardiorespiratory support, renal support, hepatic support, and areas under development such as immune support.

Indications

ECLS is indicated for acute cardiopulmonary failure with high mortality/morbidity unresponsive to maximal medical treatment and with expected organ recovery. The premise is that patients can be supported with ECLS while native function improves, either by allowing natural development or improvement (lung maturation and surfactant development), by application of medical or surgical therapies, or by transplantation. Identification of the patients that can benefit from ECLS can be challenging.

Three clinical measurement systems have been developed and tested to assist in identifying patients who will benefit from ECLS support.

$$\text{Oxygenation Index (OI)} = (MAP \times F_iO_2 \times 100)/P_aO_2$$

where *MAP* is mean airway pressure. This index has been evaluated[22,23] and has shown that an *OI* greater than 40 in 3 to 5 postductal gases was predictive of a mortality risk of 80% or greater.[24]

$$\text{Postductal alveolar-arterial oxygen gradient } [(A - a)Do_2]$$

An $(A - a)Do_2$ of 610 torr or greater despite 8 hours of maximal medical therapy predicted a mortality of 79%.[23]

$$\text{Ventilation Index} = (\text{Respiratory rate} \times Paco_2 \times \text{Peak inspiratory pressure})/1000$$

Rivera and colleagues[25] found that a ventilation index greater than 40 and OI greater than 40 were associated with a 77% mortality risk, and also found that the combination of peak inspiratory pressure of 40 cm H_2O or more and an $(A - a)Do_2$ greater than 580 mm Hg was associated with a mortality of 81%.

These clinical measurement systems are useful in quantitating the degree of cardiopulmonary derangement, and subsequently categorize patients into candidates for ECLS therapy or continued maximal medical therapy. However, the decision to initiate ECLS therapy is often a clinical decision based on clinical judgment and the patient's individual response to maximal medical therapy. Patients are commonly started on ECLS therapy when they have failed maximal medical support, significant barotrauma is imminent, and they are thought to have good potential for complete organ recovery.

The total number of neonatal ECLS runs for respiratory and cardiac failure is demonstrated in **Fig. 1**; note the increased frequency in cardiac failure cases. The survival of neonatal respiratory cases is illustrated in **Fig. 2**, and the most common diagnoses are listed in **Table 2**. The survival of neonatal cardiac cases is shown in **Fig. 3**, and the most common diagnoses are listed in **Table 3**.

Classic Contraindications and Possible Treatment Expansion

The classic contraindications to ECLS therapy are listed here. As ECLS treatment evolves and technology advances, many of the classic contraindications to ECLS are being challenged.

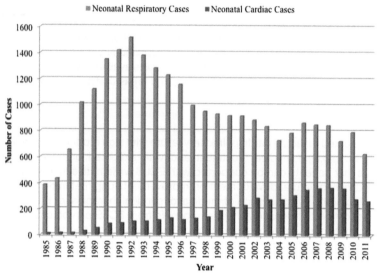

Fig. 1. Neonatal ECMO cases.

1. *EGA less than 34 weeks.* The higher incidence of intracranial bleeding in premature infants has historically precluded the use of ECLS in neonates of less than 34 weeks EGA.[26,27] However, recent data indicate that ECLS can potentially be used in infants as young as 29 weeks EGA with acceptable survival and intracranial hemorrhage (ICH) rates. Ideally development of a nonthrombogenic coating of circuit components would obviate systemic heparinization and decrease the risk of using ECLS in premature infants.[28–31]

2. *ICH greater than grade II.* Neonates with ICH of higher grades are at increased risk of extension of their hemorrhage with systemic heparinization. Although this remains true today, the development of technologies that obviate heparinization

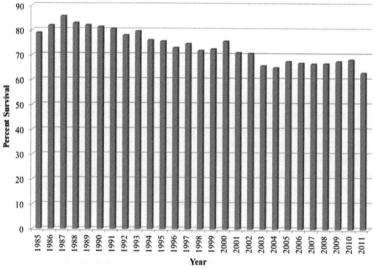

Fig. 2. Survival (%) of neonatal ECMO respiratory cases.

Table 2
Neonatal ECMO respiratory cases: survival by diagnosis

Primary Diagnosis	Total Cases	Survival (n)	Survival (%)
CDH	6376	3233	51
MAS	7825	7333	94
PPHN/PFC	4222	3265	77
Infant RDS	1511	1272	84
Sepsis	2654	1979	75
Other	2983	1887	63

Abbreviations: CDH, congenital diaphragmatic hernia; MAS, meconium aspiration syndrome; PFC, persistent fetal circulation; PPHN, persistent pulmonary hypertension of the newborn; RDS, respiratory distress syndrome.

may allow the use of ECLS in neonates with preexisting ICH in the future.[29,31–35] In addition, experience has suggested that ECMO can be applied when expected mortality is higher in neonates with grade II ICH. In such a setting, lower levels of anticoagulation are cautiously applied.

3. *Mechanical ventilation for longer than 7 to 10 days.* Mechanical ventilation classically has been associated with higher incidence of bronchopulmonary dysplasia and irreversible fibroproliferative lung disease. The duration of pre-ECMO mechanical ventilation is being challenged; data from the ELSO registry demonstrate survival of 50% to 60% after pre-ECLS mechanical ventilation of up to 14 days.[36]

4. *Cardiac arrest that requires cardiopulmonary resuscitation (CPR).* Many centers now consider patients who suffer pre-ECLS cardiac arrest candidates for support. Survival rates of up to 60% have been demonstrated in neonates who suffer cardiac arrest before or during cannulation.[37,38]

5. *Conditions incompatible with meaningful life after therapy: profound neurologic impairment, congenital anomalies, or other conditions.* With improvement in

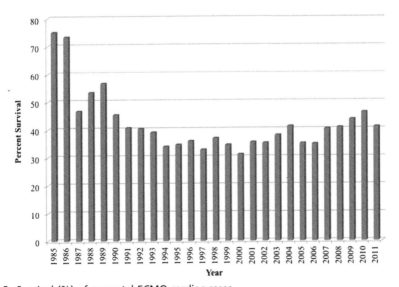

Fig. 3. Survival (%) of neonatal ECMO cardiac cases.

Table 3
Neonatal ECMO cardiac cases: survival by diagnosis

Primary Diagnosis	Total Cases	Survival (n)	Survival (%)
Congenital defect	4149	1575	38
Cardiac arrest	71	18	25
Cardiogenic shock	68	27	40
Cardiomyopathy	113	69	61
Myocarditis	55	27	49
Other	412	175	42

medical and surgical care, conditions once thought to be nonsurvivable require constant reassessment.

Outcomes

Today, ECMO is a part of routine management in the neonatal intensive care unit (ICU). Overall survival is 85%, with 98% survival for meconium aspiration and 55% survival for diaphragmatic hernia.[1] As illustrated in **Fig. 2**, overall survival after ECLS for neonatal respiratory failure has recently declined. There are likely a few reasons for this decrease in survival. Since its peak in 1992 of 1500 cases, ECLS has been used with less frequency for critically ill neonates. The lower number of cases is due to an improvement in other modalities of support such as inhaled nitric oxide, high-frequency oscillatory ventilation, and surfactant therapy. To some extent, these improvements have been realized as a result of lessons learned from early ECMO experience.[1,39–41] As a result, the neonatal patients receiving ECLS as the initial form of therapy for cardiopulmonary failure are declining, and the patients who ultimately require ECLS are probably more ill and further along the timeline of their illness.

Modalities

ECLS aims to provide perfusion of warmed, arterialized blood into the patient.[42,43] Traditionally venovenous (VV) support has been used for respiratory failure while venoarterial (VA) support has been used in cases of cardiac or combined cardiopulmonary failure. VV-ECLS can be performed through 1-site or 2-site cannulation. Traditionally blood was drained through a cannula placed in the right internal jugular (IJ) vein and returned through the femoral vein, although this approach proved problematic in newborns with small femoral veins. More recently 1-site or venovenous double-lumen (VVDL) cannulation has emerged as the preferred cannulation technique. In this mode, a single cannula is placed in the right IJ vein. Deoxygenated blood is drained from one port, pumped through the ECLS circuit where gas exchange occurs, and returned through a separate port on the same cannula into the right atrium. VA-ECLS provides complete cardiopulmonary support. Typically a drainage cannula is placed in the right IJ. Deoxygenated blood is pumped through the ECMO circuit and returned through a cannula in the right carotid artery. Historically VA-ECLS has been used more than VV-ECLS in the support of neonates. However, data from the ELSO registry demonstrate that the use of VV-ECLS is increasing for neonatal cardiopulmonary failure.[43]

ECMO II

The first generation of ECMO support devices (known as ECMO I) were used from 1975 to 2008. However, problems with the oxygenator membrane, rotational pump, and cannulae limited expansion of the technology. Recently there has been substantial technological improvement in ECMO system components and circuitry, defined as ECMO II.[44]

Modern hollow-fiber oxygenators have several advantages over the original silicon-membrane oxygenators.[45–47] The hollow-fiber design provides a much lower resistance across the oxygenator membrane, allowing for the use of centrifugal pumps in the ECMO circuit. The centrifugal pumps used now consist of a rotating impeller that spins on a small bearing or is magnetically suspended.[48] Some of the newest pumps available provide pulsatile flow.[49] In addition, the advent of the double-lumen Avalon cannula (Avalon Elite; Avalon Laboratories, Rancho Dominguez, CA, USA) allows the percutaneous placement of a single cannula for VV-ECMO support that both drains and reinfuses blood to allow for effective circuit flow.[50,51] Further-more, there has been significant research effort toward improving the biocompatibility of circuit surface-blood interfaces.[32,33] Finally, the simplification of operating the ECMO II system makes it such that a trained ICU nurse can manage the circuit, thus decreasing manpower use, as a single ECMO technician may now oversee several patients at once. These advancements provide translational development in the application and expansion of ECMO support for neonatal cardiopulmonary failure.

NOVEL USES OF ECMO
Ex utero intrapartum therapy to ECMO

Ex utero intrapartum therapy (EXIT) was originally developed for the controlled reversal of fetal tracheal occlusion in fetuses with severe congenital diaphragmatic hernia (CDH) who were treated with in utero fetal clipping or obstruction.[52] The EXIT procedure involves maintaining an infant on uteroplacental support during delivery to maximize stability.[53–56] Advances in prenatal diagnosis and the increased stability of infants during the procedure have led to the expansion of its uses to the treatment of neonates with suspected airway compromise and those who are predicted to have a particularly difficult postnatal resuscitation. Current indications for the EXIT procedure include congenital high-airway obstruction syndrome, large neck masses, large thoracic masses such as congenital pulmonary airway malformations, unilateral pulmonary agenesis, severe CDH, severe congenital cardiac anomalies, and requirement of ECMO cannulation for any of these other problems associated with cardiopulmonary compromise.[57–62] In particularly high-risk EXIT procedures, ECMO is often available in the room or is planned as an intervention after securing the airway or proceeding with further procedures. The goal of EXIT to ECMO is to avoid hypoxia, acidosis, hemodynamic instability, and prolonged resuscitation in an infant who might otherwise rapidly decompensate once off placental support.[53] **Box 1** lists the conditions for which one might consider EXIT to ECMO.[56,59]

EXIT to ECMO has been most frequently performed for infants with severe CDH, defined by liver herniation into the chest and/or pulmonary hypoplasia with low lung/head circumference ratio (LHR). Groups have performed EXIT to ECMO with LHR less than 1.4 or less than 1.0, but with current treatment outcomes for CDH the authors would only consider the highest-risk patients with an LHR less than 1.[53,56,59] Kunisaki and colleagues[59] published the largest experience with EXIT to ECMO used to treat neonates with severe CDH. Their criteria included liver herniation with an LHR less than 1.4, percentage of predicted lung volume less than 15, and/or congenital heart disease. The reported overall survival after EXIT to ECMO was 64%, which the investigators compared with a study reporting aggregate data from other centers that reported a survival rate of 52% in neonates with severe CDH who required ECMO. However, in a more recent, as yet unpublished, series of EXIT to ECMO cases for severe CDH, the same group found poorer survival than in their initial report and no

---

Box 1
Conditions to consider ECMO in conjunction with EXIT

Severe CDH

    LHR <1.0

    Liver herniation into the chest

    PPLV <15%

Severe congenital heart disease

    Severe aortic stenosis

    Hypoplastic left heart syndrome with a restrictive atrial septum

Giant congenital pulmonary airway malformations

Abbreviations: LHR, lung/head circumference ratio; PPLV, percentage of predicted lung volume.

---

clear survival benefit to the procedure (Stoffan and colleagues, unpublished data; presented at the American Academy of Pediatrics National Conference, 2011).

Late-term fetuses with severe congenital heart disease may also be treated with EXIT to ECMO. Patients with severe aortic stenosis or hypoplastic left heart syndrome with a restrictive atrial septum may be placed on VA-ECMO before ligating the umbilical cord to prevent cardiorespiratory collapse at birth. These patients are subsequently taken to the cardiac catheterization laboratory for further interventions. Neonates with thoracic masses resulting in severe pulmonary hypoplasia can be placed on ECMO if ventilatory failure develops after lung resection during the EXIT procedure.[58,60]

EXIT to ECMO has its greatest utility in late-term fetuses with anticipated cardiac or pulmonary failure at birth. However, the rarity of these cases makes it difficult to study the overall efficacy and benefit of EXIT to ECMO over standard treatment. In addition, the parameters for the use of ECMO at the time of the EXIT procedure must be more clearly defined before it can become a more widely accepted practice.

ECMO in Premature Neonates

Previous studies have shown poor survival with the use of ECMO in premature neonates. The early report by Bartlett and colleagues[15] of ECLS in 45 moribund neonates revealed a 55% survival rate for neonates overall. Nine of these patients were less than 35 weeks EGA, and 2 survived (22%). All 6 who died had ICH. A later report showed similarly worrisome survival for premature neonates less than 35 weeks EGA, namely 33% (3/15). One of these had an ICH and survived, but the other 12 patients with ICH died.[23] A study examining intracranial hemorrhage in patients on ECLS showed that all 8 of the patients less than 35 weeks EGA had an ICH, and that 6 of these died immediately after termination of ECLS while 2 died within 1 year of age.[26] Given these poor survival rates (22%–33%) and the extremely high rate of ICH (75%–100%), Cilley and colleagues[26] recommended that use of ECLS be contraindicated in neonates of less than 35 weeks EGA. However, examination of the ELSO database between 1988 and 1991 found that survival had improved to 63%, and ICH rates decreased to 37% for premature neonates born at 34 weeks EGA or younger.[26,27]

The authors recently performed a comprehensive analysis of the ELSO database from 1976 to 2008. This analysis showed no statistically significant difference in the risk of intraventricular hemorrhage (IVH) in infants of 30 to 33 weeks EGA (21%) when compared with those of 34 weeks EGA (17%), $P = .195$.[63] The overall survival rate of 54% and ICH rate of 18% for the entire cohort of neonates on ECLS at 34 weeks EGA or younger suggest that the incidence of both mortality and ICH have decreased over time, with a more dramatic reduction observed in ICH. Although the survival for the 29- to 33-week EGA group was significantly decreased (48%) when compared with those patients with EGA 34 weeks (58%, $P = .011$), one could argue that these rates are clinically acceptable. Patients born at younger EGA are expected to have a more difficult hospital course. These data suggest that ECLS in the modern era should be explored at EGA as low as 29 weeks, with reasonable survival and acceptable rates of ICH.

ARTIFICIAL PLACENTA
Rationale for an Artificial Placenta

ECMO is increasingly effective for late preterm to term infants (34–40 weeks EGA), and it might be beneficial for some infants who are 29 to 34 weeks EGA. However, a different paradigm is required for ECLS in extremely low gestational age newborns (ELGANs, 24–29 weeks EGA). ELGANs are at the greatest risk for death and poor long-term outcomes.[64–66] In particular, respiratory failure in premature neonates contributes to significant mortality and long-term disability. Conventional mechanical ventilation is often inadequate to provide gas exchange and can cause trauma to the underdeveloped lungs. Even more advanced strategies developed to minimize the trauma of conventional ventilation, including surfactant replacement therapy, nitric oxide inhalation, and high-frequency oscillatory ventilation, may at times be insufficient to support these most fragile infants.[67,68] In theory, the most effective solution is to create an artificial placenta (AP) that maintains fetal circulation and obviates mechanical ventilation and resultant devastating barotrauma by completely bypassing the lungs.

Definition of the Artificial Placenta

1. Maintenance of fetal circulation and the intrauterine environment
2. No mechanical ventilation
3. Simulated fetal breathing with fluid-filled lungs
4. A novel form of a pump-driven VV or AV ECLS/ECMO with outflow via the right jugular vein or umbilical artery, respectively, and inflow via the umbilical vein.

History of the Artificial Placenta

Research into the AP started in the 1950s as a method to treat neonatal respiratory distress. The first human study by Westin and colleagues[69] in 1958 made use of a pump-driven AV-ECLS circuit in previable fetuses, with blood drained from the umbilical artery and returned through the umbilical vein, mimicking natural fetoplacental support. As in later animal work, all fetuses were maintained in a warm artificial amniotic fluid bath. The success of this foray into human research was limited, paving the way for the laboratory study of fetal and neonatal animal models, mainly goats, sheep, and dogs. One of the first sets of animal publications on the AP was by Callaghan and colleagues from 1961 to 1965,[70–73] who reported survival of premature lambs for up to 165 minutes on AP support. Zapol, Griffith, Alexander, and others[74–77] continued to publish work on the AP for another decade, with the greatest reported success by Zapol and colleagues,[75] who reported support of an exteriorized fetus for 55 hours in 1969. The primary outcome measure in these studies was survival time, but the physiologic effects of AV-ECLS on fetal flows, gas exchange, and cerebral blood flow were not well examined. A single human study that came from this work was published in 1971 by White and colleagues,[78] who reported placing 3 premature infants on VV-ECLS using the umbilical vein for reinfusion. These babies lived for 10, 3, and 2 days with good gas-exchange parameters, but all died of bleeding due to excessive heparinization.

Successes in conventional ECMO for the treatment of neonatal respiratory failure and advances in neonatal pulmonary therapy caused work on the AP to be largely abandoned by 1980.[2,79,80] With increasing study in fetal surgery in the 1990s, several groups resumed AP research to care for those infants with respiratory failure who are too premature to be treated by conventional means. In the early 1990s, the Kuwabara group published a series of articles regarding the methodology associated with extrauterine incubation of goat fetuses after umbilical-vessel cannulation, with survival up to 10 days.[81,82] Unno and colleagues[83,84] then went on to report the support of goat fetuses using an AV-ECLS AP for up to 3 weeks. Building on this work, Yasufuku and colleagues[85] demonstrated ongoing fetal lung growth and maturation while on extrauterine AV-ECLS AP support in 1997. Despite this success, no human clinical trials of AP support were conducted, and only one report on the use of the umbilical vein as an ECMO reinfusion vessel in 4 premature infants has been published in the modern era by Kato and colleagues,[86] in 1998.

Current Artificial Placenta Research

A drawback of earlier AP circuits is the high-resistance oxygenator and high priming volumes needed for traditional ECMO circuits. The authors' group and others have attempted to investigate a pumpless system that would use a low-resistance oxygenator and decreased priming volumes.[87–89] However, umbilical artery vasospasm and circuit resistance made necessary a pump to overcome the problem of persistent hypotension and hypoperfusion (Mychaliska GB, unpublished data, 2010). Once a pump was deemed necessary, the authors postulated that VV-ECLS with right jugular drainage would provide more stable hemodynamics and serve as a better configuration for the AP.

A VV-ECLS AP offers several potential advantages over an AV-ECLS system. First, it eliminates the use of arterial vessels that are prone to spasm. Placing a cannula in the right atrium through the jugular vein allows for a passive drainage process that reduces potential negative pressure and cavitation in the circuit. In addition, VV-ECLS uses the subject's own venous system as a blood reservoir, instead of requiring an external blood reservoir. Another potential advantage relates to the drainage cannula itself. Although it is feasible to advance a large cannula (10F–12F) through the umbilical artery into the aorta in preterm sheep, this is not possible in premature human infants because of the size of the umbilical artery and vessel anatomy. It would be very difficult to place even a 6F cannula through the umbilical artery of a premature human baby. On the other hand, a larger cannula (6F–8F) can be inserted into the right IJ vein in premature infants to allow for adequate drainage. Third, a VV-ECLS AP operates in parallel with the systemic circulation. Similar to traditional VV-ECMO circuits, the fetal heart would experience little increased resistance and afterload from the parallel circuit.[43] Conversely, an AV-ECLS system with an oxygenator placed in series has the potential to increase stress on the fetal heart and contribute to cardiac failure.[90]

The authors subsequently developed a reproducible fetal sheep model of VV-ECLS, draining blood from the right jugular vein and reinfusing it through the umbilical vein. Lambs were maintained in a warm artificial amniotic bath (**Fig. 4**). The method first demonstrated long-term support (>24 hours, n = 5) with stable gas exchange and hemodynamics (**Figs. 5 and 6**).[91] However, in this set of experiments the amniotic bath became easily infected and created the problem of sepsis in animals that lived longer than 24 hours. Thus, the authors

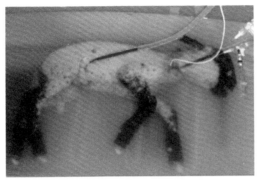

Fig. 4. Fetal lamb on VV-ECLS artificial placenta support submerged in an amniotic bath.

began maintaining experimental animals in an incubator with an amniotic fluid-filled endotracheal tube, rather than submerged in an amniotic-fluid bath (**Fig. 7**).

The authors' next set of experiments demonstrated that the VV-ECLS AP could stabilize and recover moribund fetal sheep with ventilatory failure after delivery (unpublished data). These animals had stable hemodynamics, gas exchange, and cerebral perfusion for longer than 70 hours on the AP, with a maximum of 92 hours in one animal. Lung histology at 24 hours and 77 hours on the AP demonstrated no significant difference from controls in most subjects, and despite maintaining activated clotting times between 180 and 225 seconds, there was no evidence of gross or microscopic intracerebral hemorrhage. The next steps will be aimed toward invasively and noninvasively monitoring the effect of the AP on fetal blood flow. Ongoing AP research by other groups is focused on refining AV-ECLS systems, studying fetal neurologic activity on the AP, and development of pumpless circuits.[88,92–94]

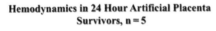

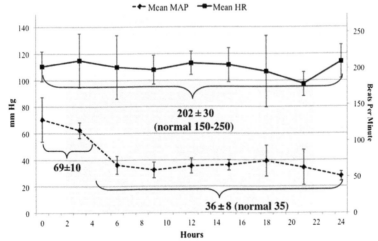

*Error bars indicate Standard Deviation

Fig. 5. Hemodynamics in 24-hour artificial placenta survivors (N = 5). HR, heart rate; MAP, mean arterial pressure.

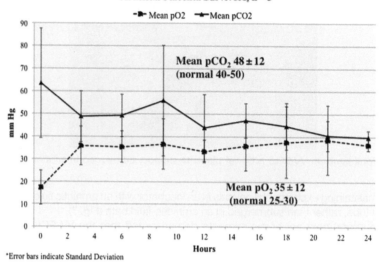

Fig. 6. Carotid arterial blood gas values in 24-hour artificial placenta survivors (N = 5). pCO$_2$, partial pressure of carbon dioxide; pO$_2$, partial pressure of oxygen.

Clinical Prognostic Factors

The ideal patient population to benefit from the AP are ELGANs (<29 weeks EGA) who fail the most aggressive pulmonary therapies, such as low peak pressure ventilation, nitric oxide inhalation, surfactant administration, and high-frequency oscillatory ventilation. Early identification of those with the highest mortality risk has been validated in this population using mortality prediction tools (CRIB II and SNAPPE II), based on data obtained in the first 12 hours of life.[95–97] In the authors' institutional experience, 483 ELGANs were treated at the University of Michigan between 2000 and 2010. The overall mortality among ELGANs was 28.8%, which predictably decreased with increasing gestational age (**Table 4**). These data are comparable to summary statistics extracted from the Vermont Oxford Network and recently published outcomes data in ELGANs treated in Boston.[98] Early identification of these infants offers the opportunity for early intervention with novel

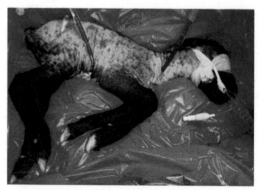

Fig.7. Fetal lamb on VV-ECLS artificial placenta support with an amniotic fluid-filled endotracheal tube.

Table 4
University of Michigan mortality in ELGANs, 2000 to 2010

	Gestational Age (wk)						
	22	23	24	25	26	27	Total ELGANs
	n = 4	n = 38	n = 103	n = 94	n = 106	n = 138	N = 483
Mortality (%)	75	55.3	43.7	27.7	22.6	14.5	28.8

Abbreviation: ELGANs, extremely low gestational age newborns.

therapies, such as the AP, to improve outcomes and elicit the greatest overall impact on prematurity-related morbidity and mortality in this highest risk group of neonates.

Potential Complications and Current Limitations

There are several potential complications and questions that must be addressed in the laboratory before the AP can be taken to the clinical setting. The first, and most pressing, is the issue of anticoagulation and the risk of ICH or IVH. Issues with IVH were the main driving force for limiting conventional ECMO to late-gestation newborns.[27,78] However, many of these reports were from a time before activated clotting time was routinely followed in systematically anticoagulated neonates, leading to excessive anticoagulation. More recent studies on the pathogenesis of IVH suggest that many causes may be iatrogenic. The mechanism of injury may be due to either a disruption of cerebral blood flow or injury to the relatively weak endothelial tissue of the germinal matrix.[99,100] Disruption of cerebral blood flow can be caused by transfusion, rapid volume expansion, or through positive pressure ventilation that may greatly increase cerebral perfusion pressures.[99,101] Avoiding ventilation and providing stable hemodynamics and gas exchange might afford the same protection against IVH. Nevertheless, to further minimize the risk of IVH, the authors propose the eventual use of nonthrombogenic surfaces in the form of biomaterials that release nitric oxide, to completely eliminate the need for anticoagulation.[29,31,34,35]

Additional research questions and areas of exploration in the development of a clinically applicable AP involve nearly every organ system and include the following:

1. Monitoring cerebral blood flow and neurologic activity
2. Evaluation of fetal blood flow and cardiac function using noninvasive means (echocardiography)
3. Further studies into lung maturation and development on AP support
4. Development of protocols for weaning off AP support to conventional ventilation or room air
5. Optimizing neonatal nutrition and metabolic balance
6. Maintaining renal and hepatic function
7. Maintaining sterility to prevent sepsis over days to weeks of support
8. Extending AP studies to extremely low gestation age animal models (600–1000 g), as all animal studies to date have used late-term fetuses (2.5–5 kg)
9. Optimizing pump, oxygenator, and circuit function.

REFERENCES

1. Bartlett RH. Extracorporeal life support: history and new directions. Semin Perinatol 2005;29:2–7.

2. Bartlett RH, Gazzaniga AB, Jefferies MR, et al. Extracorporeal membrane oxygenation (ECMO) cardiopulmonary support in infancy. Trans Am Soc Artif Intern Organs 1976;22:80–93.

3. Duyndam A, Ista E, Houmes RJ, et al. Invasive ventilation modes in children: a systematic review and meta-analysis. Crit Care 2011;15:R24.

4. Finer NN, Barrington KJ. Nitric oxide for respiratory failure in infants born at or near term. Cochrane Database Syst Rev 2006;4:CD000399.

5. Field D, Elbourne D, Hardy P, et al. Neonatal ventilation with inhaled nitric oxide vs. ventilatory support without inhaled nitric oxide for infants with severe respiratory failure born at or near term: the INNOVO multicentre randomised controlled trial. Neonatology 2007;91:73–82.

6. El Shahed AI, Dargaville P, Ohlsson A, et al. Surfactant for meconium aspiration syndrome in full term/near term infants. Cochrane Database Syst Rev 2007;3: CD002054.

7. Stevens TP, Harrington EW, Blennow M, et al. Early surfactant administration with brief ventilation vs. selective surfactant and continued mechanical ventilation for preterm infants with or at risk for respiratory distress syndrome. Cochrane Database Syst Rev 2007;3:CD003063.

8. Greenough A, Dimitriou G, Prendergast M, et al. Synchronized mechanical ventilation for respiratory support in newborn infants. Cochrane Database Syst Rev 2008;1:CD000456.

9. Mugford M, Elbourne D, Field D. Extracorporeal membrane oxygenation for severe respiratory failure in newborn infants. Cochrane Database Syst Rev 2008;3:CD001340.

10. Itoh H, Ichiba S, Ujike Y, et al. Extracorporeal membrane oxygenation following pediatric cardiac surgery: development and outcomes from a single center experience. Perfusion 2012;27(3):225–9.

11. Gibbon JH Jr. Application of a mechanical heart and lung apparatus to cardiac surgery [passim]. Minn Med 1954;37:171–85.

12. Lillehei CW, Cohen M, Warden HE, et al. The results of direct vision closure of ventricular septal defects in eight patients by means of controlled cross circulation. Surg Gynecol Obstet 1955;101:446–66.

13. Hill JD, O'Brien TG, Murray JJ, et al. Prolonged extracorporeal oxygenation for acute post-traumatic respiratory failure (shock-lung syndrome). Use of the Bramson membrane lung. N Engl J Med 1972;286:629–34.

14. Bartlett RH, Gazzaniga AB, Fong SW, et al. Prolonged extracorporeal cardiopulmonary support in man. J Thorac Cardiovasc Surg 1974;68:918–32.

15. Bartlett RH, Andrews AF, Toomasian JM, et al. Extracorporeal membrane oxygenation for newborn respiratory failure: forty-five cases. Surgery 1982;92:425–33.

16. Bartlett RH, Roloff DW, Cornell RG, et al. Extracorporeal circulation in neonatal respiratory failure: a prospective randomized study. Pediatrics 1985;76:479–87.

17. O'Rourke PP, Crone RK, Vacanti JP, et al. Extracorporeal membrane oxygenation and conventional medical therapy in neonates with persistent pulmonary hypertension of the newborn: a prospective randomized study. Pediatrics 1989;84:957–63.

18. Toomasian JM, Snedecor SM, Cornell RG, et al. National experience with extracorporeal membrane oxygenation for newborn respiratory failure. Data from 715 cases. ASAIO Trans 1988;34:140–7.

19. Zwischenberger JB, Bartlett RH, Extracorporeal Life Support Organization. ECMO: extracorporeal cardiopulmonary support in critical care. 2nd edition. Ann Arbor (MI): Extracorporeal Life Support Organization; 2000.

20. Schumacher RE, Roloff DW, Chapman R, et al. Extracorporeal membrane oxygenation in term newborns. A prospective cost-benefit analysis. ASAIO J 1993;39:873–9.

21. UK collaborative randomised trial of neonatal extracorporeal membrane oxygenation. UK Collaborative ECMO Trail Group. Lancet 1996;348:75–82.

22. Stolar CJ, Snedecor SM, Bartlett RH. Extracorporeal membrane oxygenation and neonatal respiratory failure: experience from the extracorporeal life support organization. J Pediatr Surg 1991;26:563–71.

23. Bartlett RH, Gazzaniga AB, Toomasian J, et al. Extracorporeal membrane oxygenation (ECMO) in neonatal respiratory failure. 100 cases [Erratum appears in Ann Surg 1987;205(1):11 Note: Corwin AG [corrected to Coran AG]]. Ann Surg 1986;204:236–45.

24. Ortega M, Ramos AD, Platzker AC, et al. Early prediction of ultimate outcome in newborn infants with severe respiratory failure. J Pediatr 1988;113:744–7.

25. Rivera RA, Butt W, Shann F. Predictors of mortality in children with respiratory failure: possible indications for ECMO. Anaesth Intensive Care 1990;18:385–9.

26. Cilley RE, Zwischenberger JB, Andrews AF, et al. Intracranial hemorrhage during extracorporeal membrane oxygenation in neonates. Pediatrics 1986;78:699–704.

27. Hirschl RB, Schumacher RE, Snedecor SN, et al. The efficacy of extracorporeal life support in premature and low birth weight newborns. J Pediatr Surg 1993; 28:1336–40 [discussion: 1341].

28. Meinhardt JP, Annich GM, Miskulin J, et al. Thrombogenicity is not reduced when heparin and phospholipid bonded circuits are used in a rabbit model of extracorporeal circulation. ASAIO J 2003;49:395–400.

29. Annich GM, Meinhardt JP, Mowery KA, et al. Reduced platelet activation and thrombosis in extracorporeal circuits coated with nitric oxide release polymers. Crit Care Med 2000;28:915–20.

30. Frost MC, Reynolds MM, Meyerhoff ME. Polymers incorporating nitric oxide releasing/generating substances for improved biocompatibility of blood-contacting medical devices. Biomaterials 2005;26:1685–93.

31. Zhang H, Annich GM, Miskulin J, et al. Nitric oxide-releasing fumed silica particles: synthesis, characterization, and biomedical application. J Am Chem Soc 2003;125:5015–24.

32. Major TC, Brant DO, Burney CP, et al. The hemocompatibility of a nitric oxide generating polymer that catalyzes S-nitrosothiol decomposition in an extracorporeal circulation model. Biomaterials 2011;32:5957–69.

33. Major TC, Brant DO, Reynolds MM, et al. The attenuation of platelet and monocyte activation in a rabbit model of extracorporeal circulation by a nitric oxide releasing polymer. Biomaterials 2010;31:2736–45.

34. Skrzypchak AM, Lafayette NG, Bartlett RH, et al. Effect of varying nitric oxide release to prevent platelet consumption and preserve platelet function in an in vivo model of extracorporeal circulation. Perfusion 2007;22: 193–200.

35. Wu B, Gerlitz B, Grinnell BW, et al. Polymeric coatings that mimic the endothelium: combining nitric oxide release with surface-bound active thrombomodulin and heparin. Biomaterials 2007;28:4047–55.

36. Lewis DA, Gauger P, Delosh TN, et al. The effect of pre-ECLS ventilation time on survival and respiratory morbidity in the neonatal population. J Pediatr Surg 1996;31:1110–4 [discussion: 4–5].

37. von Allmen D, Ryckman FC. Cardiac arrest in the ECMO candidate. J Pediatr Surg 1991;26:143–6.

38. del Nido PJ, Dalton HJ, Thompson AE, et al. Extracorporeal membrane oxygenator rescue in children during cardiac arrest after cardiac surgery. Circulation 1992;86:II300–4.
39. Clark RH, Huckaby JL, Kueser TJ, et al. Low-dose nitric oxide therapy for persistent pulmonary hypertension: 1-year follow-up. J Perinatol 2003;23:300–3.
40. Christou H, Van Marter LJ, Wessel DL, et al. Inhaled nitric oxide reduces the need for extracorporeal membrane oxygenation in infants with persistent pulmonary hypertension of the newborn. Crit Care Med 2000;28:3722–7.
41. Clark RH, Kueser TJ, Walker MW, et al. Low-dose nitric oxide therapy for persistent pulmonary hypertension of the newborn. Clinical Inhaled Nitric Oxide Research Group. N Engl J Med 2000;342:469–74.
42. Bartlett RH. Extracorporeal life support for cardiopulmonary failure. Curr Probl Surg 1990;27:621–705.
43. Skinner SC, Hirschl RB, Bartlett RH. Extracorporeal life support. Semin Pediatr Surg 2006;15:242–50.
44. MacLaren G, Combes A, Bartlett RH. Contemporary extracorporeal membrane oxygenation for adult respiratory failure: life support in the new era. Intensive Care Med 2012;38:210–20.
45. Khoshbin E, Roberts N, Harvey C, et al. Poly-methyl pentene oxygenators have improved gas exchange capability and reduced transfusion requirements in adult extracorporeal membrane oxygenation. ASAIO J 2005;51:281–7.
46. Nishinaka T, Tatsumi E, Katagiri N, et al. Up to 151 days of continuous animal perfusion with trivial heparin infusion by the application of a long-term durable antithrombogenic coating to a combination of a seal-less centrifugal pump and a diffusion membrane oxygenator. J Artif Organs 2007;10:240–4.
47. Peek GJ, Killer HM, Reeves R, et al. Early experience with a polymethyl pentene oxygenator for adult extracorporeal life support. ASAIO J 2002;48:480–2.
48. Mendler N, Podechtl F, Feil G, et al. Seal-less centrifugal blood pump with magnetically suspended rotor: rot-a-flot. Artif Organs 1995;19:620–4.
49. Talor J, Yee S, Rider A, et al. Comparison of perfusion quality in hollow-fiber membrane oxygenators for neonatal extracorporeal life support. Artif Organs 2010;34:E110–6.
50. Wang D, Zhou X, Liu X, et al. Wang-Zwische double lumen cannula-toward a percutaneous and ambulatory paracorporeal artificial lung. ASAIO J 2008; 54:606–11.
51. Bermudez CA, Rocha RV, Sappington PL, et al. Initial experience with single cannulation for venovenous extracorporeal oxygenation in adults. Ann Thorac Surg 2010;90:991–5.
52. Mychaliska GB, Bealer JF, Graf JL, et al. Operating on placental support: the ex utero intrapartum treatment procedure. J Pediatr Surg 1997;32:227–30 [discussion: 30–1].
53. Liechty KW. Ex-utero intrapartum therapy. Semin Fetal Neonatal Med 2010;15: 34–9.
54. Hirose S, Harrison MR. The ex utero intrapartum treatment (EXIT) procedure. Semin Neonatol 2003;8:207–14.
55. Hedrick HL. Ex utero intrapartum therapy. Semin Pediatr Surg 2003;12:190–5.
56. Marwan A, Crombleholme TM. The EXIT procedure: principles, pitfalls, and progress. Semin Pediatr Surg 2006;15:107–15.
57. Hedrick HL, Flake AW, Crombleholme TM, et al. The ex utero intrapartum therapy procedure for high-risk fetal lung lesions. J Pediatr Surg 2005;40: 1038–43 [discussion: 44].

58. Mychaliska GB, Bryner BS, Nugent C, et al. Giant pulmonary sequestration: the rare case requiring the EXIT procedure with resection and ECMO. Fetal Diagn Ther 2009;25:163–6.

59. Kunisaki SM, Barnewolt CE, Estroff JA, et al. Ex utero intrapartum treatment with extracorporeal membrane oxygenation for severe congenital diaphragmatic hernia. J Pediatr Surg 2007;42:98–104 [discussion: 6].

60. Kunisaki SM, Fauza DO, Barnewolt CE, et al. Ex utero intrapartum treatment with placement on extracorporeal membrane oxygenation for fetal thoracic masses. J Pediatr Surg 2007;42:420–5.

61. Bouchard S, Johnson MP, Flake AW, et al. The EXIT procedure: experience and outcome in 31 cases. J Pediatr Surg 2002;37:418–26.

62. Liechty KW, Crombleholme TM, Flake AW, et al. Intrapartum airway management for giant fetal neck masses: the EXIT (ex utero intrapartum treatment) procedure. Am J Obstet Gynecol 1997;177:870–4.

63. Kim A, Erickson K, Rana A, et al. Pushing the boundaries of ECLS: outcomes in <34 week EGA neonates. Puerto Rico: American Pediatric Surgical Association; 2009.

64. Markestad T, Kaaresen PI, Ronnestad A, et al. Early death, morbidity, and need of treatment among extremely premature infants. Pediatrics 2005;115:1289–98.

65. Behrman RE, Adashi EY, Allen MC, et al. Preterm birth: causes, consequences, and prevention. Washington, DC: Institute of Medicine of the National Academics; 2006.

66. Hack M, Fanaroff AA. Outcomes of children of extremely low birthweight and gestational age in the 1990s. Semin Neonatol 2000;5:89–106.

67. Rimensberger PC. Neonatal respiratory failure [review]. Curr Opin Pediatr 2002; 14(3):315–21.

68. Ventre KM, Arnold JH. High frequency oscillatory ventilation in acute respiratory failure [review]. Paediatr Respir Rev 2004;5(4):323–32.

69. Westin B, Nyberg R, Enhorning G. A technique for perfusion of the previable human fetus. Acta Paediatr 1958;47(4):339–49.

70. Callaghan JC, Angeles J, Boracchia B, et al. Studies of the first successful delivery of an unborn lamb after 40 minutes in the artificial placenta. Can J Surg 1963;6:199–205.

71. Callaghan JC, Maynes EA, Hug HR. Studies on lambs of the development of an artificial placenta. Review of nine long-term survivors of extracorporeal circulation maintained in a fluid medium. Can J Surg 1965;8:208–13.

72. Callaghan JC, Angeles JD. Long term extracorporeal circulation in the development of an artificial placenta for respiratory distress of the newborn. Surg Forum 1961;12:215–7.

73. Callaghan JC, Angeles JD, Boracchia B, et al. Studies in the development of an artificial placenta the possible use of long-term extracorporeal circulation for respiratory distress of the newborn. Circulation 1963;XXVII:686–90.

74. Griffith BP, Borovetz HS, Hardesty RL, et al. Arteriovenous ECMO for neonatal respiratory support. A study in perigestational lambs. J Thorac Cardiovasc Surg 1979;77(4):595–601.

75. Zapol WM, Kolobow T, Pierce Jevurek GG, et al. Artificial placenta: two days of total extrauterine support of the isolated premature lamb fetus. Science 1969; 166:617–8.

76. Chamberlain G. An artificial placenta: the development of an extracorporeal system for maintenance of immature infants with respiratory problems. Am J Obstet Gynecol 1968;100(5):615–26.

77. Alexander DP, Britton HG, Nixon DA. Maintenance of sheep fetuses by an extra-corporeal circuit for periods up to 24 hours. Am J Obstet Gynecol 1968;102(7): 969–75.

78. White JJ, Andrews HG, Risemberg H, et al. Prolonged respiratory support in newborn infants with a membrane oxygenator. Surgery 1971;70:288–96.

79. Touch SM, Shaffer TH, Greenspan JS. Managing our first breaths: a reflection on the past several decades of neonatal pulmonary therapy. Neonatal Netw 2002; 21:13–20.

80. Halliday HL. History of surfactant from 1980. Biol Neonate 2005;87:317–22.

81. Kuwabara Y, Okai T, Imanishi Y, et al. Development of extrauterine fetal incuba-tion system using extracorporeal membrane oxygenator. Artif Organs 1987; 11(3):224–7.

82. Kuwabara Y, Okai T, Kozuma S, et al. Artificial placenta: long-term extrauterine incubation of isolated goat fetuses. Artif Organs 1989;13(6):527–31.

83. Unno N, Kuwabara Y, Okai T, et al. Development of an artificial placenta: survival of isolated goat fetuses for three weeks with umbilical arteriovenous extracorpo-real membrane oxygenation. Artif Organs 1993;17:996–1003.

84. Unno N, Kuwabara Y, Shinozuka N, et al. Development of artificial placenta: oxygen metabolism of isolated goat fetuses with umbilical arteriovenous extra-corporeal membrane oxygenation. Fetal Diagn Ther 1990;5(3-4):189–95.

85. Yasufuku M, Hisano K, Sakata M, et al. Arterio-venous extracorporeal membrane oxygenation of fetal goat incubated in artificial amniotic fluid (artificial placenta): influence on lung growth and maturation [see comment]. J Pediatr Surg 1998; 33:442–8.

86. Kato J, Nagaya M, Niimi N, et al. Venovenous extracorporeal membrane oxygenation in newborn infants using the umbilical vein as a reinfusion route. J Pediatr Surg 1998;33:1446–8.

87. Reoma JL, Rojas A, Kim AC, et al. Development of an artificial placenta I: pump-less arterio-venous extracorporeal life support in a neonatal sheep model. J Pe-diatr Surg 2009;44:53–9.

88. Arens J, Schoberer M, Lohr A, et al. NeonatOx: a pumpless extracorporeal lung support for premature neonates. Artif Organs 2011;35:997–1001.

89. Awad JA, Cloutier R, Fournier L, et al. Pumpless respiratory assistance using a membrane oxygenator as an artificial placenta: a preliminary study in newborn and preterm lambs. J Invest Surg 1995;8(1):21–30.

90. Seo T, Ito T, Iio K, et al. Experimental study on the hemodynamic effects of veno-arterial extracorporeal membrane oxygenation with an automatically driven blood pump on puppies. Artif Organs 1991;15:402–7.

91. Gray BW, El-Sabagh A, Rojas-Pena A, et al. Development of an artificial placenta IV: 24 hour venovenous extracorporeal life support in premature lambs. ASAIO J 2012;58:148–54.

92. Pak SC, Song CH, So GY, et al. Extrauterine incubation of fetal goats applying the extracorporeal membrane oxygenation via umbilical artery and vein. J Korean Med Sci 2002;17:663–8.

93. Sakata M, Hisano K, Okada M, et al. A new artificial placenta with a centrifugal pump: long-term total extrauterine support of goat fetuses. J Thorac Cardiovasc Surg 1998;115:1023–31.

94. Kozuma S, Nishina H, Unno N, et al. Goat fetuses disconnected from the placenta, but reconnected to an artificial placenta, display intermittent breathing movements. Biol Neonate 1999;75(6):388–97.

95. Richardson DK, Corcoran JD, Escobar GJ, et al. SNAP-II and SNAPPE-II: Simplified newborn illness severity and mortality risk scores. J Pediatr 2001; 138:92–100.
96. Parry G, Tucker J, Tarnow-Mordi W, et al. an update of the clinical risk index for babies score. Lancet 2003;361:1789–91.
97. Carvalho PR, Moreira ME, Sa RA, et al. SNAPPE-II application in newborns with very low birth weight: evaluation of adverse outcomes in severe placental dysfunction. J Perinat Med 2011;39:343–7.
98. Tyson JE, Parikh NA, Langer J, et al. Intensive care for extreme prematurity—moving beyond gestational age. N Engl J Med 2008;358:1672–81.
99. Milligan DW. Failure of autoregulation and intraventricular haemorrhage in preterm infants. Lancet 1980;1:896–8.
100. Tarby TJ, Volpe JJ. Intraventricular hemorrhage in the premature infant. Pediatr Clin North Am 1982;29:1077–104.
101. Goldberg RN, Chung D, Goldman SL, et al. The association of rapid volume expansion and intraventricular hemorrhage in the preterm infant. J Pediatr 1980;96:1060–3.

Congenital Lung Lesions

Pramod S. Puligandla, MD, MSc, FRCSC[a],
Jean-Martin Laberge, MD, FRCSC[b],*

KEYWORDS

- Congenital cystic adenomatoid malformation
- Congenital pulmonary airway malformation • Bronchial atresia • Lung sequestration
- Pleuropulmonary blastoma • Thoracoscopic surgery • Fetal diagnosis and treatment
- Compensatory lung growth

KEY POINTS

- The congenital cystic adenomatoid malformation volume ratio is a useful tool to predict which congenital lung lesions will lead to fetal hydrops.
- Maternal betamethasone administration may have a therapeutic effect for large echogenic fetal lung lesions causing hydrops.
- Less invasive fetal treatment options have proven successful in selected instances of symptomatic congenital lung lesions.
- Bronchial atresia is increasingly recognized as the underlying cause of many congenital lung lesions.
- Pleuropulmonary blastoma type I may be diagnosed prenatally, is a de novo tumor rather than a malignant transformation of a preexisting cystic lung lesion and cannot be distinguished from type I and IV congenital pulmonary airway malformation based on imaging.
- Long-term observational studies are under way to clarify the natural history of congenital lung lesions.

PRENATAL DIAGNOSIS AND TREATMENT

Great strides have been made in the last 2 decades in the understanding of congenital lung lesions (CLLs), especially when diagnosed prenatally. Although 15 to 20 years ago an early report demonstrated that 40% of CLLs were lethal in utero[1] and some centers were recommending pregnancy termination simply because of mediastinal shift or polyhydramnios, most investigators now agree that the majority of pregnancies with an affected fetus can be carried with an excellent outcome.[2–7]

The authors have no relevant commercial relationships to disclose.
[a] Pediatric Surgery, Montreal Children's Hospital, McGill University Health Center, McGill University, 2300 Tupper Street, Suite C-811, Montreal, Quebec H3P 1P3, Canada; [b] Pediatric Surgery, Montreal Children's Hospital, McGill University Health Center, McGill University, 2300 Tupper Street, Suite C-820, Montreal, Quebec H3H 1P3, Canada
* Corresponding author.
E-mail address: jean-martin.laberge@muhc.mcgill.ca

Clin Perinatol 39 (2012) 331–347
doi:10.1016/j.clp.2012.04.009
0095-5108/12/$ – see front matter © 2012 Elsevier Inc. All rights reserved.

Fetal lung lesions are usually divided into macrocystic, microcystic (echogenic), and mixed lesions based on their sonographic appearance.[8,9] Many ultrasonographers incorrectly try to classify anomalies as congenital cystic adenomatoid malformations (CCAMs) according to Stocker type I, II, or III, which is a classification based not only on postnatal cyst size but also on histology.[10] The presence of a systemic arterial supply to the abnormal lung is generally thought to be associated with lung sequestration, either intralobar (ILS) or extralobar sequestration (ELS), but many examples of hybrid lesions, with features of CCAM and sequestration, have been described.[3,8,11] Other lesions that are part of the differential diagnosis include bronchial atresia, which is recognized with increasing frequency and may be the underlying pathologic condition common to many apparently distinct lesions; congenital lobar overinflation; and bronchogenic cysts.[11–14] Congenital lobar or segmental emphysema has been described with increasing frequency in recent years.[15–18] The lesion is usually hyperechoic/microcystic on prenatal ultrasonography, fluid-filled on initial postnatal imaging, and becomes hyperlucent with time. Some of these characteristics may be related to bronchial atresia, and changes compatible with CCAM may be found in the resected specimen.[13,19] Only the postnatal evolution and sometimes, the histologic evaluation can provide a definitive diagnosis (**Fig. 1**).[2] The terms *congenital lung lesion* or *congenital lung malformation* should therefore be used as a generic name prenatally instead of trying to make a histologic diagnosis. The size (anteroposterior, laterolateral, and craniocaudal), volume, location, appearance, presence of a systemic arterial supply, mediastinal shift, presence of pleural effusion, ascites, and other signs of hydrops should be given to complete the ultrasonography report. In some instances when the diagnosis is unclear, fetal magnetic resonance imaging may be useful.[11,20,21]

Fetuses developing hydrops because of a large mass or high flow from a systemic artery have a worse prognosis (**Fig. 2**),[5,9] and when this happens in the second trimester, fetal intervention is warranted. For cystic lesions, repeated cyst aspiration may be a temporizing measure (**Fig. 3**), but cyst reexpansion occurs within 24 to 72 hours. Thoracoamniotic shunting has been used successfully in many centers to drain large cystic lung lesions and hydrothoraces associated with sequestrations.[4,9,22,23] In addition to the risks of bleeding, membrane separation, and preterm labor, chest wall deformities have recently been described in association with shunt placement before 21 weeks' gestation.[24] For solid lesions, fetal lobectomy has been practiced successfully in a few centers.[9,25–27] Others have tried less invasive methods, such as radiofrequency or laser ablation, with limited success[28,29] although laser was recently used to successfully ablate the feeding artery of pulmonary sequestrations causing hydrops.[30,31] Percutaneous ultrasound-guided sclerotherapy has also been described in 3 cases each of CCAM and ILS[32,33] and a single case of ELS.[34] If the 100% success rate in these small reports can be duplicated by other groups, this simple and inexpensive technique may prove to be most useful and widely applicable around the world.

Because many CLLs appear to regress in utero[35] whereas others progress to hydrops, a prognostic tool that allows closer monitoring of fetuses at risk was developed.[36] The CCAM volume ratio (CVR) measures the volume of the lung lesion, divided by the head circumference to normalize for gestational age. In the initial reports, a CVR of greater than 1.6 in echogenic lesions was associated with an increased risk of hydrops. Others have found the cutoff at a CVR of greater than 2.0.[27]

An exciting development in the prenatal management of large echogenic lung lesions is the finding that maternal betamethasone administration may lead to regression of the lesion and reversal of hydrops. The initial observation was made in

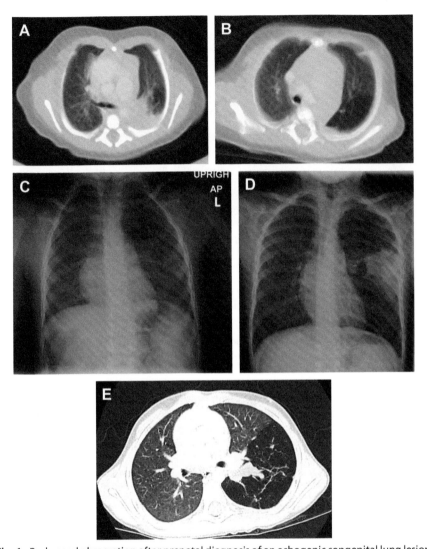

Fig. 1. Prolonged observation after prenatal diagnosis of an echogenic congenital lung lesion. (*A*) Postnatal computed tomography (CT) at 9 days of age shows fluid retention in the posterior segment of the right upper lobe (RUL), which becomes hyperlucent on CT repeated at 3 months (*B*). This remains stable on CT at 6 months. He was transferred to our center at 18 months of age because of constipation related to repair of a low imperforate anus repair. With a presumed diagnosis of congenital lobar/segmental emphysema and in the absence of symptoms, the patient was observed. A chest radiograph at 2 years showed mild hyperlucency in the RUL (*C*); this was stable 2 years later. At 5 years, he developed recurrent respiratory tract infections and a chest radiograph showed segmental consolidation in the RUL (*D*), which resolved after antibiotic treatment. Increased hyperlucency is seen on CT 4 months later (*E*). Thoracoscopic left upper lobectomy was difficult because of inflammation and a fused fissure, and the patient developed a postoperative hydropneumothorax requiring chest tube reinsertion and readmission to hospital. Pathology was consistent with type II CCAM, without evidence of bronchial atresia, but changes suggestive of bronchomalacia. However, an atresia that would have been at the bronchial staple line cannot be excluded. (*From* Harrison MR, Albanese CT, Hawgood SP, et al. Fetoscopic temporary tracheal occlusion by means of detachable balloon for congenital diaphragmatic hernia. Am J Obstet Gynecol 2001;185:732; with permission.)

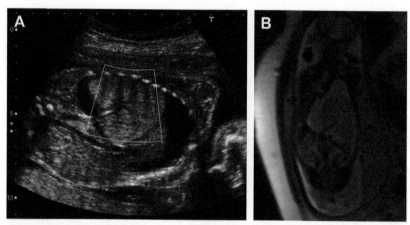

Fig. 2. (*A*) Fetal ultrasonography with Doppler at 24 weeks' gestation, showing an echogenic lung mass with a large systemic artery from the aorta, initially seen at 18 weeks' gestation. The lesion had progressed to hydrothorax and some ascites as seen on this magnetic resonance image done a few days later (*B*). Mediastinal shift with a compressed right lung (*arrow*) and the abnormal systemic artery (*asterisk*) are apparent. The mother declined fetal intervention and the fetus died 2 weeks later.

patients with fetal hydrops who were in the second trimester and not candidates for fetal intervention.[37] A variable but definite response has since been observed by several groups.[38–40]

A final development in the prenatal management of large CLLs causing a significant and prolonged mediastinal shift with a high likelihood of pulmonary hypoplasia is the ex utero intrapartum treatment (EXIT) procedure, with resection of the abnormal lobe while on placental bypass.[41] Although an 89% of survival was achieved in high-risk patients in 1 center, the superiority of this more invasive approach over standard postnatal resection remains to be confirmed. An EXIT-to-extracorporeal membrane oxygenation approach has also been advocated, with delayed lung resection.[42]

POSTNATAL CLASSIFICATION OF CLLs

The most common clinically relevant CLL is known as CCAM, which was classified into 3 types in 1977 by Stocker,[10] who later changed the nomenclature to congenital pulmonary airway malformation (CPAM) and expanded it to 5 types by adding types 0 and IV.[43] Not only is there overlap between the clinical, imaging, and histopathological features of the various types, but also there are many hybrid lesions, for example typical ELS or ILS with a systemic arterial supply and histologic features of CPAM. This findings have led several pathologists to question whether CCAM/CPAM is an entity on its own or simply represents changes in the developing lung caused by an insult such as bronchial atresia.[14,44,45] Langston classifies CLLs into bronchopulmonary malformations, pulmonary hyperplasia, and other cystic lesions (**Box 1**).[44] Although not perfect, this classification emphasizes the various combinations and overlap observed between these malformations. What is not clear from the table but stated clearly in Langston's review, is that most bronchial atresia specimens demonstrate parenchymal maldevelopment consistent with CCAM type II, and conversely, most CCAM type II are associated with bronchial atresia if specifically sought, an observation supported by other pediatric pathologists.[13,14] The authors have

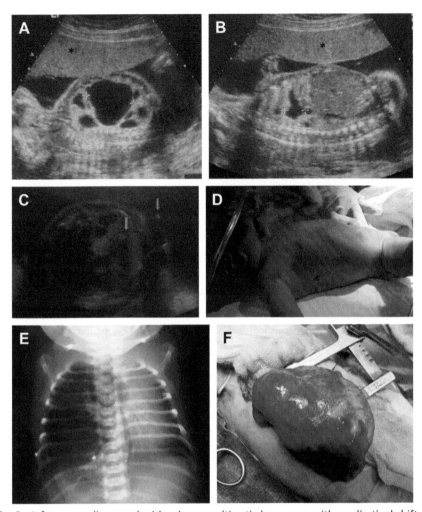

Fig. 3. A fetus was diagnosed with a large multicystic lung mass with mediastinal shift at 18 weeks' gestation (*A*). Serial ultrasonography revealed early signs of hydrops at 21 weeks; because of an anterior placenta (*asterisk*), initial management consisted of needle decompression twice weekly and the hydrops resolved. All cysts were decompressed by single-needle thoracentesis (*B*). At 27 weeks' gestation, a thoracoamniotic shunt (*arrows*) was placed and provided decompression until term (*C*). The baby was delivered vaginally at term and did not require intubation. The shunt was still in place (*D*) and was covered with a sterile plastic bag connected to a Heimlich valve. The chest radiograph showed significant mediastinal shift (*E*); therefore, the baby was operated immediately despite having minimal symptoms. The massive right upper lobe enlargement can be seen at surgery (*F*). Pathology showed type I CCAM. (Fetal pictures *Courtesy of* Dr Samir Khalifé, Department of Obstetrics and Gynecology, Royal Victoria Hospital, Montreal, Quebec, Canada.)

previously demonstrated the multiple facets of pulmonary sequestration.[46] In fact, there are multiple facets to all types of CLLs.

Other recent attempts at changing or simplifying the nomenclature of CLL have failed. The authors agree with Sebire[47] that Achiron's[8,48] suggestion to change the unpopular malinosculation terminology[49] to fetal lung dysplasia was ill-advised. Similarly, the

---

Box 1
Classification of CLLs

Bronchopulmonary malformation

    Bronchogenic cyst (noncommunicating bronchopulmonary foregut malformation)

    Bronchial atresia

        Isolated

        With systemic arterial/venous connection (ILS)

        With connection to gastrointestinal tract (ILS/complex or communicating bronchopulmonary foregut malformation)

        Systemic arterial connection to normal lung

    Cystic adenomatoid malformation, large cyst type (Stocker type 1)

        Isolated

        With systemic arterial/venous connection (hybrid lesion/ILS)

    Cystic adenomatoid malformation, small cyst type (Stocker type 2)

        Isolated

        With systemic arterial/venous connection (hybrid lesion/ILS)

    ELS

        Without connection to gastrointestinal tract (with/without cystic adenomatoid malformation, smell cyst type)

        With connection to gastrointestinal tract (complex/communicating bronchopulmonary foregut malformation)

Pulmonary hyperplasia and related lesions

    Laryngeal atresia

    Solid or adenomatoid cystic adenomatoid malformation (Stocker type 3)

    Polyalveolar lobe

Congenital lobar overinflation

Other cystic lesions

    Lymphatic/lymphangiomatous cysts

    Enteric cysts

    Mesothelial cysts

    Simple parenchymal cysts

    Low-grade cystic pleuropulmonary blastoma

From Langston C. New concepts in the pathology of congenital lung malformations. Semin Pediatr Surg 2003;12:17–37; with permission.

---

terminology *congenital thoracic malformation* proposed by Bush[50,51] seems too broad and would include chest wall deformities such as Poland Syndrome, rib fusions, and mesenchymal hamartoma, as well as pericardial cysts, thymic masses and other malformations unrelated to lung development. The authors conclude that CLL or congenital lung malformation are the best terms to use in a fetus, neonate, or older child, until surgical and pathologic findings provide more definite information. Foregut duplication cysts (bronchogenic or esophageal) situated in the mediastinum represent one of the subtypes more easily diagnosed with imaging; they are included in the classification even though they are not lung malformations per se.[52,53] The term bronchopulmonary foregut malformation (BPFM) is also valid but is more often used in the context of communicating BPFMs.[46]

CLLs AND MALIGNANCY

Two types of malignancies have been linked to CLL: (1) sarcomas/blastomas are found in infants and young children and have now been regrouped under the term *pleuropulmonary blastomas* (PPBs), and (2) bronchioloalveolar carcinomas (BACs) are seen in adolescents and young adults. The link between type I CPAM leading to mucinous BAC is well established both by multiple case reports highlighting malignancy development in incompletely resected CPAM and the molecular/premalignant aspect of the mucinous cells seen in type I CPAM.[2,54-58] The risk of malignant transformation of type I CPAM has been estimated to be approximately 1%.[54] The BAC associated with CPAM appears at a younger age than regular BAC (a single report in an infant, 6 others in children 6 to 11 years old, and the rest in teenagers and young adults) and tends to have a more indolent course but can be lethal, justifying complete surgical resection early in life.[54,59-61]

As far as the transformation of congenital cystic lung lesions into sarcoma-type malignancies in infancy, it is now believed that most of these reports represent de novo PPB.[62,63] After the efforts of Priest and colleagues[64] to establish a registry to study this rare neoplasm of infancy, it has become recognized that most untreated PPBs progress from the cystic type I to the solid type III, via a mixed type II. Type I PPB is indistinguishable radiologically from types I and IV CPAM, and even pathologic differentiation from the latter may be difficult (**Fig. 4**).[63,65-68] There are even reports of prenatally diagnosed cystic lung lesions, which proved to be PPB, and the authors' case is yet another example (see **Fig. 4**).[69,70] The diagnosis of PPB should be strongly suspected in the presence of (or family history of) multifocal or bilateral lung cysts, spontaneous pneumothorax in infants, or young children with lung cysts, renal cysts or cystic nephroma, intestinal polyps, thyroid hyperplasia, sarcomas, gonadal, and other tumors. As stated by Priest, even though "40% of PPB patients manifest some familial or constitutional clue to finding PPB, there remain about 60% of PPB cases without a prior hint of malignancy. A child diagnosed with early cystic PPB has a significantly better prognosis than those in whom solid tumor has emerged."[63] Although the prevalence of CCAM/CPAM has been estimated at 1 in 15,000 to 1 in 25,000 births,[35,71] PPB is rare with less than 500 cases reported.[2,63] Another recent report estimates the respective prevalences of CCAM and PPB at 1 in 12,000 and 1 in 250,000 live births, with a 4% risk of PPB in apparently benign cystic lung malformation.[72]

POSTNATAL MANAGEMENT
Operation or Observation?

Although the management of children with symptomatic congenital lung malformations is reasonably straightforward, there is ongoing debate regarding the need for, and the timing of, surgical intervention in children with asymptomatic lesions. The arguments for and against observation have been previously described[2] and are predominantly based on small retrospective experiences and indirect evidence. Those who support surgery for cystic lung malformations and ILS worry mostly about the development of infection during the period of observation. Other reasons why surgery has been advocated include the uncertainty in the diagnosis based on radiology alone

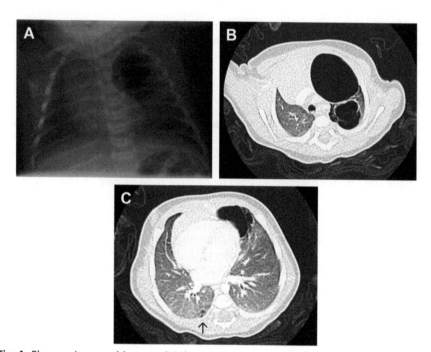

Fig. 4. Pleuropulmonary blastoma (PPB). A cystic mass was seen in the left upper thorax at 21 weeks' gestation. (*A*) Two weeks after birth the child is asymptomatic but on chest radiograph a large cystic air-filled lesion is seen; the cyst enlarged significantly at 4 weeks, prompting a CT scan at 5 weeks. A large cyst with smaller cysts was seen in the left upper lobe (*B*), as well as tiny cysts in the right lower lobe (*C, arrow*). Even though the radiological appearance was consistent with large cyst CCAM, because of the preoperative suspicion of PPB, a thoracotomy was favored to thoracoscopic resection. This confirmed a macrocystic lesion in the left upper lobe, sparing the lingula, but a left upper lobectomy was performed. Pathology showed a type I PPB with negative margins. The result of an abdominal ultrasonography was normal, and the DICER1 mutation was absent in the patient.[113] No adjuvant chemotherapy was administered given the young age (2 months), and the child remains well 2 years later. CT was repeated at 19 months of age and showed resolution of the small right lower lobe lucencies. The case was submitted to the PPB registry. (The authors thank Dr Sherif Emil for permission to include his patient.)

(see previous discussions on CPAM type I/IV and PPB; **Fig. 4**), the discordance between the presumptive radiological and final pathologic diagnosis,[73] the risk of pneumothorax and delayed malignant transformation, and the basic contention that these lesions do not represent variants of normal and thus should be removed.[2,73–78] Despite the above arguments, the need for surgery is not a universally held opinion. Chetcuti and Crabbe,[79] in a simple letter to the editor, stated that they followed up more than 100 children with antenatally diagnosed CLL. From this group, approximately 10% showed neonatal symptoms and underwent surgery, approximately 5% developed lower respiratory tract infections during early childhood, and the remaining are under follow-up and remain symptom-free.[79] These results are supported by preliminary observations, also reported only as a letter to the editor in the same journal and issue, from the LoTOS study (Long Term Outcome Study) from University College London, UK, where 52 of 90 patients have been prospectively observed without complications.[80] Although the authors were unable to find an update of these studies in a proper peer-reviewed publication since 2006, some investigators have cited them to support conservative management.[81]

For those who support surgical intervention for CLLs, the safety of pulmonary resection in infants and children is no longer a source of debate. Complication rates after surgery range between 6% and 9% and are mostly related to air leak. Mortality is a very rare occurrence in experienced hands.[73,81] The vast majority of these infants are also extubated immediately after the procedure,[73] which may be facilitated by the use of regional/epidural anesthesia.[82] Two small prospective studies involving 19[83] and 28 patients,[84] respectively, have also demonstrated that most infants who had pulmonary resection in infancy have normal pulmonary function on long-term follow-up.

The timing of surgery also remains controversial. Proponents of early intervention cite the risk of developing infection or cardiorespiratory symptoms (eg, respiratory distress, pneumothorax) as the main reasons to pursue an early operative strategy.[6,73,74,82,85,86] Most individuals would delay the surgery until after 2 to 3 months of age to decrease anesthetic risks and the need for postoperative ventilatory support.[2,73,82,87–89] The risk of infection for CLLs has been estimated to range between 10% and 30% within the first year of life,[2,90] thus potentially making any surgical resection more difficult.[91] Indeed, some reports have documented that 20% to 86% of asymptomatic patients will develop symptoms,[74,81,92] often by 6 months of age.[86] The significance of operating on symptomatic patients should not be underestimated.[74,93,94] In 1 retrospective study examining 45 infants who underwent surgery at a mean age of 3.8 months, infants who were symptomatic had significantly more intraoperative and postoperative complications as well as longer hospitalizations compared with infants who were asymptomatic at the time of operation.[82] Other studies have contested these findings, citing no apparent difference in outcomes for those children who were observed for a period of time before surgery versus those who underwent earlier intervention, even if symptoms did develop during the period of observation.[81,90,95] Some investigators recommend early surgical resection, which takes advantage of the compensatory lung growth in the early months of life.[2,73,82,83,88,96–98] Other investigators articulate a more skeptical position. For example, Naito and colleagues,[84] did not observe a correlation between age at lobectomy and pulmonary function in 28 prospectively followed infants who had pulmonary resections at a mean age of 13 months (range 3 days–56 months). These investigators subsequently discounted compensatory lung growth as a valid reason to support early surgical resection. However, Beres and colleagues,[83] in a slightly smaller prospective series of 19 infants who underwent surgery at a mean age of 4.7 months (range 3 days–9 months) and were followed for more than 5 years postoperatively reported that 86% had normal lung function compared with population norms. Eight of the 19 infants were old enough to have lung volumes measured, all of whom had normal or increased total lung capacity (TLC). The ratio of residual volume (RV) to TLC was normal (<30%) in 6 infants and increased in 2 infants. These results suggest that compensatory lung growth occurs in most patients because the RV to TLC ratio would have been increased if lung growth occurred by alveolar distension alone. It is possible that the impact of compensatory lung growth in the study by Naito and colleagues[84] may have been confounded by the older age at lobectomy. Furthermore, Komori and colleagues,[99] have also supported the existence of compensatory lung growth based on their results. In their study, radionuclide scanning demonstrated fewer emphysematous changes and reduced RV to TLC ratios in the 8 infants undergoing surgery at less than 1 year of age versus older children. The debate regarding the indications for surgery and its timing compared with simple observation will continue until long-term outcome studies involving large numbers of patients can be completed. The LoTOS study[80] may provide us with this opportunity, but long-term follow-up into adulthood is necessary to fully assess the risk of delayed complications such as infection, pneumothorax, and BAC. Furthermore, risks related to repeated radiological studies including computed tomography (CT) will have to be taken into account.[100] Based on the current uncertainty regarding the natural history of these lesions, informed consent must include detailed discussions that describe both surgical and conservative/observation strategies and the current state of evidence.

Surgical Options: Segmental Resection Versus Lobectomy; Thoracotomy Versus Thoracoscopy

Open thoracotomy has been the traditional standard for the resection of CLLs. Some surgeons have advocated for segmentectomy for these lesions,[101] even by thoracoscopy.[102] Parenchymal sparing operations have an intuitive appeal in the young growing child, but the risks and consequences of incomplete resection,[2] which may only be identified after final pathology review or on postoperative CT scanning, may make this approach more applicable for smaller well-defined lesions.[102] Many investigators recommend lobectomy to prevent postoperative air leaks, residual disease, and late malignancy.[74,87,88] In a recent systematic review, nonanatomic resections were associated with a 15% rate of residual disease, compared with 0% with lobectomy.[95] Segmental resections should be reserved for very localized malformations (such as small ILSs) and for the rare patients with multilobar or bilateral involvement. Lobectomy is also preferred for pulmonary lesions where PPB is considered in the differential diagnosis.

The emergence of advanced minimally invasive techniques has led to the increasing use of thoracoscopy for CLL. Albanese and colleagues,[103] were the first to describe the successful use of thoracoscopic resection in 14 infants with a mean age of 6 months. Subsequently, Albanese and Rothenberg,[75] in one of the largest experiences to date, reported on 144 consecutive thoracoscopic lobectomies in patients aged 2 days to 18 years. Only 1 patient in this series required conversion to open thoracotomy, and the average length of stay for patients was 2.8 days. Several other reports have also described the feasibility and safety of thoracoscopic lung resections.[104–107] The common trends among these reports include longer operative times yet significantly shorter lengths of stay compared with traditional open techniques. Neonatal thoracoscopic lobectomy has also been shown to be associated with minimal morbidity. Rothenberg and colleagues,[105] described their experience in 75 patients weighing less than 10 kg who had prenatally diagnosed CLLs, a much more challenging subset of patients because of their smaller size. The technique involved the use of three or four, 3- to 5-mm valved ports, a 5-mm curved dissector, a vascular sealing device, and single-lung ventilation. Thoracic insufflation to 4 to 6 mm Hg was also maintained without cardiorespiratory consequences. Only 1 patient in this series required conversion to open thoracotomy due to bleeding complications. Although all patients received tube thoracostomies, the mean length of stay was only 2.4 days, which was shorter by 1 to 2 days compared with their historical experience with open thoracotomy. These results have been supported by others groups around the world with conversion rates ranging from 0% to 14%.[108–112] However, a theme that has emerged is the impact of previous clinical and/or subclinical infection on the ability to complete the resection thoracoscopically. Vu and colleagues,[108] in 12 thoracoscopic cases, found a higher rate of conversion in those infants who had previous infections. Garrett-Cox and colleagues[107] also suggested that thoracoscopic resection be undertaken before the onset of symptoms or infection because 5 out of 6 patients who were previously infected required conversion to open thoracotomy.

Patients with congenital lobar emphysema/overinflation represent another subset of patients in whom a thoracoscopic approach may be more challenging.[109] From a technical standpoint, there have also been cases of instrument malfunction or thermal injury from vascular sealing devices.[110] This may have pertinent implications in those infants with adhesions and difficult dissections because of previous infection.

SUMMARY

Some of the recent advances in the management of congenital lung malformations have been presented. Prenatally, some of the most significant are

- The development of a prognostic tool (the CVR) to predict the development of hydrops.
- The discovery of a therapeutic effect of maternal betamethasone administration for large solid malformations causing hydrops.
- The use of less invasive techniques such as percutaneous laser and sclerotherapy to treat some of the life-threatening lesions.
- The confirmation of the usefulness of more invasive techniques such as thoracoamniotic shunts, fetal lobectomy, and EXIT procedure.

In the diagnosis and nomenclature areas, significant findings include

- The increasing awareness of the role played by bronchial atresia in the pathogenesis of many types of CLL.
- The recognition of the overlap between and coexistence of different types of CLL.
- The recognition that type I PPB may be clinically and radiologically indistinguishable from CCAM, that PPB is a de novo tumor rather than malignant degeneration of a benign cystic lesion, and that PPB may be present prenatally (see **Fig. 4**).

Postnatally, although the debate over the management of asymptomatic congenital lung malformations continues, the arguments the authors previously made favoring the resection of all cystic lung lesions remain valid and are reinforced by recent literature regarding PPB.[2] Other key points include

- Small ELSs (ie, not aerated) without significant shunting may be observed as they rarely lead to complications and they may regress spontaneously.[2]
- Asymptomatic lobar or segmental overinflation may also be observed, but the diagnosis is not always clear (see **Fig. 1**).
- Long-term observational studies are under way to clarify the natural history of CLL.
- More studies are now available confirming the safety of lung resection in infancy and demonstrating normal lung function several years postoperatively.
- Thoracoscopic resection is gaining popularity and is more easily performed in the absence of prior infection.

REFERENCES

1. Thorpe-Beeston JG, Nicolaides KH. Cystic adenomatoid malformation of the lung: prenatal diagnosis and outcome. Prenat Diagn 1994;14:677–88.
2. Laberge JM, Puligandla P, Flageole H. Asymptomatic congenital lung malformations. Semin Pediatr Surg 2005;14:16–33.
3. Adzick NS. Management of fetal lung lesions. Clin Perinatol 2003;30:481–92.

4. Davenport M, Warne SA, Cacciaguerra S, et al. Current outcome of antenally diagnosed cystic lung disease. J Pediatr Surg 2004;39:549–56.

5. Azizkhan RG, Crombleholme TM. Congenital cystic lung disease: contemporary antenatal and postnatal management. Pediatr Surg Int 2008;24:643–57.

6. Lakhoo K. Management of congenital cystic adenomatous malformations of the lung. Arch Dis Child Fetal Neonatal Ed 2009;94:F73–6.

7. Kunisaki SM, Barnewolt CE, Estroff JA, et al. Large fetal congenital cystic adenomatoid malformations: growth trends and patient survival. J Pediatr Surg 2007;42:404–10.

8. Achiron R, Hegesh J, Yagel S. Fetal lung lesions: a spectrum of disease. New classification based on pathogenesis, two-dimensional and color Doppler ultrasound. Ultrasound Obstet Gynecol 2004;24:107–14.

9. Adzick NS, Flake AW, Crombleholme TM. Management of congenital lung lesions. Semin Pediatr Surg 2003;12:10–6.

10. Stocker JT, Madewell JE, Drake RM. Congenital cystic adenomatoid malformation of the lung. Classification and morphologic spectrum. Hum Pathol 1977;8: 155–71.

11. Alamo L, Gudinchet F, Reinberg O, et al. Prenatal diagnosis of congenital lung malformations. Pediatr Radiol 2012;42(3):273–83.

12. Farrugia MK, Raza SA, Gould S, et al. Congenital lung lesions: classification and concordance of radiological appearance and surgical pathology. Pediatr Surg Int 2008;24:987–91.

13. Peranteau WH, Merchant AM, Hedrick HL, et al. Prenatal course and postnatal management of peripheral bronchial atresia: association with congenital cystic adenomatoid malformation of the lung. Fetal Diagn Ther 2008;24: 190–6.

14. Riedlinger WF, Vargas SO, Jennings RW, et al. Bronchial atresia is common to extralobar sequestration, intralobar sequestration, congenital cystic adenomatoid malformation, and lobar emphysema. Pediatr Dev Pathol 2006;9:361–73.

15. Ankermann T, Oppermann HC, Engler S, et al. Congenital masses of the lung, cystic adenomatoid malformation versus congenital lobar emphysema: prenatal diagnosis and implications for postnatal treatment. J Ultrasound Med 2004;23: 1379–84.

16. Olutoye OO, Coleman BG, Hubbard AM, et al. Prenatal diagnosis and management of congenital lobar emphysema. J Pediatr Surg 2000;35:792–5.

17. Pariente G, Aviram M, Landau D, et al. Prenatal diagnosis of congenital lobar emphysema: case report and review of the literature. J Ultrasound Med 2009; 28:1081–4.

18. Paramalingam S, Parkinson E, Sellars M, et al. Congenital segmental emphysema: an evolving lesion. Eur J Pediatr Surg 2010;20:78–81.

19. Seo T, Ando H, Kaneko K, et al. Two cases of prenatally diagnosed congenital lobar emphysema caused by lobar bronchial atresia. J Pediatr Surg 2006;41: e17–20.

20. Liu YP, Chen CP, Shih SL, et al. Fetal cystic lung lesions: evaluation with magnetic resonance imaging. Pediatr Pulmonol 2010;45:592–600.

21. Costa F, Kaganov H, O'Mahony E, et al. Diagnosis of diaphragmatic hernia with associated congenital lung lesions: contribution of fetal MRI. Fetal Diagn Ther 2011;29:111–5.

22. Knox EM, Kilby MD, Martin WL, et al. In-utero pulmonary drainage in the management of primary hydrothorax and congenital cystic lung lesion: a systematic review. Ultrasound Obstet Gynecol 2006;28:726–34.

23. Mann S, Wilson RD, Bebbington MW, et al. Antenatal diagnosis and management of congenital cystic adenomatoid malformation. Semin Fetal Neonatal Med 2007;12:477–81.
24. Merchant AM, Peranteau W, Wilson RD, et al. Postnatal chest wall deformities after fetal thoracoamniotic shunting for congenital cystic adenomatoid malformation. Fetal Diagn Ther 2007;22:435–9.
25. Adzick NS. Open fetal surgery for life-threatening fetal anomalies. Semin Fetal Neonatal Med 2010;15:1–8.
26. Phaloprakarn C, Pott Bartsch EM, Harrison MR. Residual congenital cystic adenomatoid malformation and thoracic scar deformation after fetal surgery: a case report. J Pediatr Surg 2006;41:e11–4.
27. Cass DL, Olutoye OO, Cassady CI, et al. Prenatal diagnosis and outcome of fetal lung masses. J Pediatr Surg 2011;46:292–8.
28. Bruner JP, Jarnagin BK, Reinisch L. Percutaneous laser ablation of fetal congenital cystic adenomatoid malformation: too little, too late? Fetal Diagn Ther 2000; 15:359–63.
29. Ong SS, Chan SY, Ewer AK, et al. Laser ablation of foetal microcystic lung lesion: successful outcome and rationale for its use. Fetal Diagn Ther 2006; 21:471–4.
30. Oepkes D, Devlieger R, Lopriore E, et al. Successful ultrasound-guided laser treatment of fetal hydrops caused by pulmonary sequestration. Ultrasound Obstet Gynecol 2007;29:457–9.
31. Ruano R, de A Pimenta EJ, Marques da Silva M, et al. Percutaneous intrauterine laser ablation of the abnormal vessel in pulmonary sequestration with hydrops at 29 weeks' gestation. J Ultrasound Med 2007;26:1235–41.
32. Bermudez C, Perez-Wulff J, Arcadipane M, et al. Percutaneous fetal sclerotherapy for congenital cystic adenomatoid malformation of the lung. Fetal Diagn Ther 2008;24:237–40.
33. Bermudez C, Perez-Wulff J, Bufalino G, et al. Percutaneous ultrasound-guided sclerotherapy for complicated fetal intralobar bronchopulmonary sequestration. Ultrasound Obstet Gynecol 2007;29:586–9.
34. Nicolini U, Cerri V, Groli C, et al. A new approach to prenatal treatment of extralobar pulmonary sequestration. Prenat Diagn 2000;20:758–60.
35. Laberge JM, Flageole H, Pugash D, et al. Outcome of the prenatally diagnosed congenital cystic adenomatoid lung malformation: a Canadian experience. Fetal Diagn Ther 2001;16:178–86.
36. Crombleholme TM, Coleman B, Hedrick H, et al. Cystic adenomatoid malformation volume ratio predicts outcome in prenatally diagnosed cystic adenomatoid malformation of the lung. J Pediatr Surg 2002;37:331–8.
37. Tsao K, Hawgood S, Vu L, et al. Resolution of hydrops fetalis in congenital cystic adenomatoid malformation after prenatal steroid therapy. J Pediatr Surg 2003; 38:508–10.
38. Curran PF, Jelin EB, Rand L, et al. Prenatal steroids for microcystic congenital cystic adenomatoid malformations. J Pediatr Surg 2010;45: 145–50.
39. Morris LM, Lim FY, Livingston JC, et al. High-risk fetal congenital pulmonary airway malformations have a variable response to steroids. J Pediatr Surg 2009;44:60–5.
40. Peranteau WH, Wilson RD, Liechty KW, et al. Effect of maternal betamethasone administration on prenatal congenital cystic adenomatoid malformation growth and fetal survival. Fetal Diagn Ther 2007;22:365–71.

41. Hedrick HL, Flake AW, Crombleholme TM, et al. The ex utero intrapartum therapy procedure for high-risk fetal lung lesions. J Pediatr Surg 2005;40: 1038–43 [discussion: 1044].

42. Kunisaki SM, Fauza DO, Barnewolt CE, et al. Ex utero intrapartum treatment with placement on extracorporeal membrane oxygenation for fetal thoracic masses. J Pediatr Surg 2007;42:420–5.

43. Stocker JT. Congenital pulmonary airway malformation: a new name and an expanded classification of congenital cystic adenomatoid malformations of the lung. Histopathology 2002;41:424–31.

44. Langston C. New concepts in the pathology of congenital lung malformations. Semin Pediatr Surg 2003;12:17–37.

45. Kunisaki SM, Fauza DO, Nemes LP, et al. Bronchial atresia: the hidden pathology within a spectrum of prenatally diagnosed lung masses. J Pediatr Surg 2006;41:61–5 [discussion: 61–5].

46. Bratu I, Flageole H, Chen MF, et al. The multiple facets of pulmonary sequestration. J Pediatr Surg 2001;36:784–90.

47. Sebire NJ. Fetal lung lesions: a new classification of fetal lung dysplasia. Ultrasound Obstet Gynecol 2004;24:590–1.

48. Achiron R, Zalel Y, Lipitz S, et al. Fetal lung dysplasia: clinical outcome based on a new classification system. Ultrasound Obstet Gynecol 2004; 24:127–33.

49. Clements BS, Warner JO. Pulmonary sequestration and related congenital bronchopulmonary-vascular malformations: nomenclature and classification based on anatomical and embryological considerations. Thorax 1987;42:401–8.

50. Bush A. Congenital lung disease: a plea for clear thinking and clear nomenclature. Pediatr Pulmonol 2001;32:328–37.

51. Bush A. Prenatal presentation and postnatal management of congenital thoracic malformations. Early Hum Dev 2009;85:679–84.

52. Bratu I, Laberge JM, Flageole H, et al. Foregut duplications: is there an advantage to thoracoscopic resection? J Pediatr Surg 2005;40:138–41.

53. Azzie G, Beasley S. Diagnosis and treatment of foregut duplications. Semin Pediatr Surg 2003;12:46–54.

54. West D, Nicholson AG, Colquhoun I, et al. Bronchioloalveolar carcinoma in congenital cystic adenomatoid malformation of lung. Ann Thorac Surg 2007; 83:687–9.

55. Lantuejoul S, Nicholson AG, Sartori G, et al. Mucinous cells in type 1 pulmonary congenital cystic adenomatoid malformation as mucinous bronchioloalveolar carcinoma precursors. Am J Surg Pathol 2007;31:961–9.

56. Ota H, Langston C, Honda T, et al. Histochemical analysis of mucous cells of congenital adenomatoid malformation of the lung: Insights into the carcinogenesis of pulmonary adenocarcinoma expressing gastric mucins. Am J Clin Pathol 1998;110:450–5.

57. Wang NS, Chen MF, Chen FF. The glandular component in congenital cystic adenomatoid malformation of the lung. Respirology 1999;4:147–53.

58. Stacher E, Ullmann R, Halbwedl I, et al. Atypical goblet cell hyperplasia in congenital cystic adenomatoid malformation as a possible preneoplasia for pulmonary adenocarcinoma in childhood: a genetic analysis. Hum Pathol 2004;35:565–70.

59. Ramos SG, Barbosa GH, Tavora FR, et al. Bronchioloalveolar carcinoma arising in a congenital pulmonary airway malformation in a child: case report with an update of this association. J Pediatr Surg 2007;42:E1–4.

60. Summers RJ, Shehata BM, Bleacher JC, et al. Mucinous adenocarcinoma of the lung in association with congenital pulmonary airway malformation. J Pediatr Surg 2010;45:2256–9.
61. Mani H, Shilo K, Galvin JR, et al. Spectrum of precursor and invasive neoplastic lesions in type 1 congenital pulmonary airway malformation: case report and review of the literature. Histopathology 2007;51:561–5.
62. Pai S, Eng HL, Lee SY, et al. Correction: pleuropulmonary blastoma, not rhabdomyosarcoma in a congenital lung cyst. Pediatr Blood Cancer 2007; 48:370–1.
63. Priest JR, Williams GM, Hill DA, et al. Pulmonary cysts in early childhood and the risk of malignancy. Pediatr Pulmonol 2009;44:14–30.
64. Priest JR, Hill DA, Williams GM, et al. Type I pleuropulmonary blastoma: a report from the International Pleuropulmonary Blastoma Registry. J Clin Oncol 2006;24: 4492–8.
65. Hill DA, Dehner LP, Ackerman LV, et al. A cautionary note about congenital cystic adenomatoid malformation (CCAM) type 4 (multiple letters). Am J Surg Pathol 2004;28:554–5.
66. MacSweeney F, Papagiannopoulos K, Goldstraw P, et al. An assessment of the expanded classification of congenital cystic adenomatoid malformations and their relationship to malignant transformation. Am J Surg Pathol 2003;27: 1139–46.
67. Oliveira C, Himidan S, Pastor AC, et al. Discriminating preoperative features of pleuropulmonary blastomas (PPB) from congenital cystic adenomatoid malformations (CCAM): a retrospective, age-matched study. Eur J Pediatr Surg 2011;21:2–7.
68. Al-Backer N, Puligandla PS, Su W, et al. Type 1 pleuropulmonary blastoma in a 3-year-old male with a cystic lung mass. J Pediatr Surg 2006;41:e13–5.
69. Miniati DN, Chintagumpala M, Langston C, et al. Prenatal presentation and outcome of children with pleuropulmonary blastoma. J Pediatr Surg 2006;41: 66–71.
70. Mechoulan A, Leclair MD, Yvinec M, et al. [Pleuropulmonary blastoma: a case of early neonatal diagnosis through antenatal scan screening]. Gynecol Obstet Fertil 2007;35:437–41 [in French].
71. Gornall AS, Budd JLS, Draper ES, et al. Congenital cystic adenomatoid malformation: accuracy of prenatal diagnosis, prevalence and outcome in a general population. Prenat Diagn 2003;23:997–1002.
72. Nasr A, Himidan S, Pastor AC, et al. Is congenital cystic adenomatoid malformation a premalignant lesion for pleuropulmonary blastoma? J Pediatr Surg 2010; 45:1086–9.
73. Tsai AY, Liechty KW, Hedrick HL, et al. Outcomes after postnatal resection of prenatally diagnosed asymptomatic cystic lung lesions. J Pediatr Surg 2008; 43:513–7.
74. Wong A, Vieten D, Singh S, et al. Long-term outcome of asymptomatic patients with congenital cystic adenomatoid malformation. Pediatr Surg Int 2009;25: 479–85.
75. Albanese CT, Rothenberg SS. Experience with 144 consecutive pediatric thoracoscopic lobectomies. J Laparoendosc Adv Surg Tech A 2007;17:339–41.
76. Lejeune C, Deschildre A, Thumerelle C, et al. Spontaneous pneumothorax revealing cystic adenomatoid malformation of the lung in a 13-year-old child. Pneumothorax revelateur d'une malformation adenomatoide kystique du poumon chez un enfant de 13 ans. Arch Pediatr 1999;6:863–6.

77. Metivier AC, Denoux Y, Tcherakian C, et al. [Pulmonary cystic adenomatoid malformation in an adult patient: an underdiagnosed disease]. Rev Pneumol Clin 2011;67:275–80 [in French].

78. Niimi T, Gotoh M. [Pneumothorax secondary to congenital bronchial atresia]. Kyobu Geka 2010;63:324–7 [in Japanese].

79. Chetcuti PA, Crabbe DC. CAM lungs: the conservative approach. Arch Dis Child Fetal Neonatal Ed 2006;91:F463–4.

80. Jaffe A, Chitty LS. Congenital cystic adenomatoid malformations may not require surgical intervention. Arch Dis Child Fetal Neonatal Ed 2006;91:F464.

81. Colon N, Schlegel C, Pietsch J, et al. Congenital lung anomalies: can we postpone resection? J Pediatr Surg 2012;47:87–92.

82. Aspirot A, Puligandla PS, Bouchard S, et al. A contemporary evaluation of surgical outcome in neonates and infants undergoing lung resection. J Pediatr Surg 2008;43:508–12.

83. Beres A, Aspirot A, Paris C, et al. A contemporary evaluation of pulmonary function in children undergoing lung resection in infancy. J Pediatr Surg 2011;46: 829–32.

84. Naito Y, Beres A, Lapidus-Krol E, et al. Does earlier lobectomy result in better long term pulmonary function in children with congenital lung anomalies? A prospective study. J Pediatr Surg, in press.

85. Eber E. Antenatal diagnosis of congenital thoracic malformations: early surgery, late surgery, or no surgery? Semin Respir Crit Care Med 2007;28:355–66.

86. Conforti A, Aloi I, Trucchi A, et al. Asymptomatic congenital cystic adenomatoid malformation of the lung: is it time to operate? J Thorac Cardiovasc Surg 2009; 138:826–30.

87. Khosa JK, Leong SL, Borzi PA. Congenital cystic adenomatoid malformation of the lung: indications and timing of surgery. Pediatr Surg Int 2004;20:505–8.

88. Shanmugam G, MacArthur K, Pollock JC. Congenital lung malformations–antenatal and postnatal evaluation and management. Eur J Cardiothorac Surg 2005; 27:45–52.

89. Calvert JK, Lakhoo K. Antenatally suspected congenital cystic adenomatoid malformation of the lung: postnatal investigation and timing of surgery. J Pediatr Surg 2007;42:411–4.

90. Aziz D, Langer JC, Tuuha SE, et al. Perinatally diagnosed asymptomatic congenital cystic adenomatoid malformation: to resect or not? J Pediatr Surg 2004;39:329–34 [discussion: 329–34].

91. Pelizzo G, Barbi E, Codrich D, et al. Chronic inflammation in congenital cystic adenomatoid malformations. An underestimated risk factor? J Pediatr Surg 2009;44:616–9.

92. Hammond PJ, Devdas JM, Ray B, et al. The outcome of expectant management of congenital cystic adenomatoid malformations (CCAM) of the lung. Eur J Pediatr Surg 2010;20:145–9.

93. Sueyoshi R, Okazaki T, Urushihara N, et al. Managing prenatally diagnosed asymptomatic congenital cystic adenomatoid malformation. Pediatr Surg Int 2008;24:1111–5.

94. Marshall KW, Blane CE, Teitelbaum DH, et al. Congenital cystic adenomatoid malformation: Impact of prenatal diagnosis and changing strategies in the treatment of the asymptomatic patient. Am J Roentgenol 2000;175:1551–4.

95. Stanton M, Njere I, Ade-Ajayi N, et al. Systematic review and meta-analysis of the postnatal management of congenital cystic lung lesions. J Pediatr Surg 2009;44:1027–33.

96. McBride JT, Wohl ME, Strieder DJ. Lung growth and airway function after lobectomy in infancy for congenital lobar emphysema. J Clin Invest 1980;66:962–70.
97. Frenckner B, Freyschuss U. Pulmonary function after lobectomy for congenital lobar emphysema and congenital cystic adenomatoid malformation. A follow-up study. Scand J Thorac Cardiovasc Surg 1982;16:293–8.
98. Takeda SI, Miyoshi S, Inoue M, et al. Clinical spectrum of congenital cystic disease of the lung in children. Eur J Cardiothorac Surg 1999;15:11–7.
99. Komori K, Kamagata S, Hirobe S, et al. Radionuclide imaging study of long-term pulmonary function after lobectomy in children with congenital cystic lung disease. J Pediatr Surg 2009;44:2096–100.
100. Frush DP, Donnelly LF, Rosen NS. Computed tomography and radiation risks: what pediatric health care providers should know. Pediatrics 2003;112:951–7.
101. Makhija Z, Moir CR, Allen MS, et al. Surgical management of congenital cystic lung malformations in older patients. Ann Thorac Surg 2011;91:1568–73 [discussion: 1573].
102. Johnson SM, Grace N, Edwards MJ, et al. Thoracoscopic segmentectomy for treatment of congenital lung malformations. J Pediatr Surg 2011;46:2265–9.
103. Albanese CT, Sydorak RM, Tsao K, et al. Thoracoscopic lobectomy for prenatally diagnosed lung lesions. J Pediatr Surg 2003;38:553–5.
104. Rothenberg SS. First decade's experience with thoracoscopic lobectomy in infants and children. J Pediatr Surg 2008;43:40–4 [discussion: 45].
105. Rothenberg SS, Kuenzler KA, Middlesworth W, et al. Thoracoscopic lobectomy in infants less than 10 kg with prenatally diagnosed cystic lung disease. J Laparoendosc Adv Surg Tech A 2011;21:181–4.
106. Nasr A, Bass J. Thoracoscopic versus open resection for congenital lung lesions: a meta-analysis. J Pediatr Surg, in press.
107. Garrett-Cox R, MacKinlay G, Munro F, et al. Early experience of pediatric thoracoscopic lobectomy in the UK. J Laparoendosc Adv Surg Tech A 2008;18:457–9.
108. Vu LT, Farmer DL, Nobuhara KK, et al. Thoracoscopic versus open resection for congenital cystic adenomatoid malformations of the lung. J Pediatr Surg 2008;43:35–9.
109. Rahman N, Lakhoo K. Comparison between open and thoracoscopic resection of congenital lung lesions. J Pediatr Surg 2009;44:333–6.
110. Kaneko K, Ono Y, Tainaka T, et al. Thoracoscopic lobectomy for congenital cystic lung diseases in neonates and small infants. Pediatr Surg Int 2010;26:361–5.
111. Boubnova J, Peycelon M, Garbi O, et al. Thoracoscopy in the management of congenital lung diseases in infancy. Surg Endosc 2011;25:593–6.
112. Diamond IR, Herrera P, Langer JC, et al. Thoracoscopic versus open resection of congenital lung lesions: a case-matched study. J Pediatr Surg 2007;42:1057–61.
113. Hill DA, Ivanovich J, Priest JR, et al. DICER1 mutations in familial pleuropulmonary blastoma. Science 2009;325:965.

Surgical Advances in the Fetus and Neonate: Esophageal Atresia

Shaun M. Kunisaki, MD, MSc[a],*, John E. Foker, MD, PhD[b,c]

KEYWORDS

- Esophageal atresia • Tracheoesophageal fistula • Thoracoscopic repair • Long gap

KEY POINTS

- Prenatal ultrasound findings, including an absent stomach bubble, polyhydramnios, and a dilated proximal esophageal pouch, suggest the presence of an esophageal atresia.
- At some hospitals, many patients with short-gap esophageal atresia are now candidates for thoracoscopic repair, which offers the promise of lower surgical morbidity compared to thoracotomy when performed by pediatric surgeons with expertise in advanced minimally invasive techniques.
- The management of long-gap esophageal atresia continues to be a technically challenging endeavor with several options available based on the expertise of the tertiary care referral center.
- In many infants with long-gap esophageal atresia, primary repair following tension-induced growth of the esophagus (Foker process) now serves as a viable alternative to more traditional methods of conduit reconstruction, including gastric transposition.
- Further accumulation of long-term data in patients undergoing esophageal growth induction should help clarify appropriate patient selection and enable more objective comparisons of outcomes after the different operations.

The surgical management of infants born with esophageal atresia (EA) with or without tracheoesophageal fistula (TEF) represents one of the major triumphs of pediatric surgery in the twentieth century.[1] After five failed attempts, Dr Cameron Height, a thoracic surgeon at the University of Michigan, performed the first successful primary repair of a neonate with EA/TEF in 1941.[2] Since this initial report, advances in surgical technique and neonatal care have steadily improved survival rates in babies

---

[a] Department of Surgery, Fetal Diagnosis and Treatment Center, C.S. Mott Children's and Von Voigtlander Women's Hospital, University of Michigan Medical School, 1540 East Hospital Drive, SPC 4211, Ann Arbor, MI 48109, USA; [b] Division of Cardiovascular and Thoracic Surgery, University of Minnesota Medical School, 420 Delaware Street SE, Mayo Mail Code 207, Minneapolis, MN 55455, USA; [c] Esophageal Atresia Treatment Program, Children's Hospital Boston, Harvard Medical School, 300 Longwood Avenue, Fegan 3, Boston, MA 02115, USA
* Section of Pediatric Surgery, C.S. Mott Children's Hospital, 1540 East Hospital Drive, SPC 4211, Ann Arbor, MI 48109.
E-mail address: shaunkun@umich.edu

Clin Perinatol 39 (2012) 349–361
doi:10.1016/j.clp.2012.04.007   perinatology.theclinics.com

within the EA/TEF spectrum. Based on 2006 data from a major pediatric referral center, survival of EA/TEF children with birth weights greater than 1500 g and no major cardiac anomalies is now more than more than 98%.[3]

Despite these successes, the morbidity of traditional methods of operative repair can still be significant in some patients. As a result, surgeons are continuing to refine the operative techniques used to repair EA/TEF. This article focuses on these more recent developments in treatment, including thoracoscopic repair for short-gap EA and tension-induced esophageal growth (often referred to as the *Foker process*) for long-gap EA. Although no consensus exists yet among pediatric surgeons regarding the role of these procedures in the management of EA/TEF, one can reasonably expect that as they continue to evolve, their application will become even more widespread.

EMBRYOLOGY

EA/TEF disorders occur in approximately one in 3500 live births. The malformation is caused by a complex and poorly understood process involving environmental, biomechanical, genetic, and other factors that result in abnormal foregut development during the fourth week of gestation.[4] At this stage of embryonic development, the ventral portion of the foregut gives rise to the trachea and lungs, whereas the esophagus develops from its dorsal aspect. Environmental factors that have been implicated in EA/TEF include exposure to methimazole, diethylstilbestrol, exogenous sex hormones, infectious diseases, maternal alcohol and tobacco use, maternal employment in agriculture or horticulture fields, first-trimester maternal diabetes, and advanced maternal age.[5]

Hereditary factors seem to play a minimal role in the origin of EA/TEF. The risk that a second child would be born with EA in the same family is on the order of 1%. If one twin is born with EA, there is only a 2.5% chance that the second twin will also have the anomaly.[5] Between 10% and 25% of infants with EA have three or more additional nonrandom anomalies, including vertebral, anorectal, cardiac, tracheal, esophageal, renal, and limb abnormalities, which form the VACTERL spectrum.[6] Those with isolated EA (Gross type A, **Fig. 1**B) are at highest risk for VACTERL deformities. An additional 10% of infants with EA/TEF are associated with genetic syndromes, including trisomy 18, 21, and 13. Single gene disorders that may include EA/TEF are CHARGE syndrome (*CHD7* gene), DiGeorge syndrome (*TBX1* gene), Feingold syndrome (*MYCN* gene), Opitz syndrome (*MID1* gene), Anophthalmia-Esophageal-Genital (AEG) syndrome (*SOX2* gene), and Fanconi anemia (*FACC* gene).[5]

PRENATAL DIAGNOSIS

Despite continuing advances in ultrasound imaging, the diagnosis of EA/TEF in the fetus remains difficult. Only a minority of cases are diagnosed prenatally.[7] According to several studies, between 10% and 40% of all patients with EA/TEF are identified antenatally through ultrasound.[8–10] Although the presence of anomalies within the VACTERL spectrum raises suspicion of a possible EA/TEF disorder, the most common finding suggestive of fetal EA is an absent or small stomach bubble in conjunction with polyhydramnios. Unfortunately, the sensitivity and specificity of these findings are low, and the positive predictive value for EA in the presence of an absent stomach bubble and polyhydramnios ranges between 44% and 56%.[9,11] Moreover, fetuses with an isolated EA can still have a normal-appearing, fluid-filled stomach because of the production of gastric secretions alone.[12] Based on the relatively low predictive value of fetal ultrasonography, prenatal counseling of parents in suspected EA/TEF cases should always be guarded to avoid unnecessary parental anxiety.

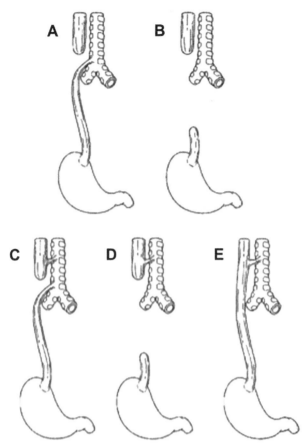

Fig. 1. (*A*) Esophageal atresia with distal tracheoesophageal fistula. (*B*) Esophageal atresia with tracheoesophageal fistula. (*C*) Esophageal atresia with proximal and distal tracheoesophageal fistula. (*D*) Esophageal atresia with proximal tracheoesophageal fistula. (*E*) Isolated tracheoesophageal fistula. (*From* Bruch SW, Coran AG. Congenital Malformations of the Esophagus. Pediatric Gastrointestinal and Liver Disease. 4th edition. Philadelphia: Elsevier; 2011. p. 222–31; with permission.)

More recent evidence suggests that the predictive value for EA may be increased if a dilated proximal esophageal pouch (upper pouch sign) is identified.[8,13] The upper pouch sign is highly specific for EA but is difficult to detect until the third trimester.[14] The role of fetal MRI in EA/TEF remains undefined but may be helpful in confirming suspected cases identified with ultrasound.[15,16] Nonimaging modalities to detect fetal EA cases have also been reported in the past several years. For example, the amniotic fluid of the fetus in EA/TEF has been shown to have higher levels of certain biochemical markers, including total protein and alpha-fetoprotein.[17] These findings have not been validated in larger studies.

Prenatally diagnosed cases of EA/TEF have been associated with slightly higher mortality rates when compared with cases diagnosed postnatally.[7,9] However, the most important predictors of overall outcome are the degree of prematurity and the presence of associated anomalies, particularly cardiac and chromosomal defects. A fetal echocardiogram and an amniocentesis for fetal karyotype analysis is indicated in suspected cases. A small but increased incidence of prematurity is seen among infants with EA/TEF when compared with the general population, most likely because of polyhydramnios from fetal esophageal obstruction. Based on an unpublished review of the last 85 patients with EA/TEF managed at the University of Michigan C.S. Mott Children's Hospital, the mean gestational age at birth was 35.7 weeks.

SHORT-GAP ATRESIA
Initial Management

Any neonate noted to have excessive oral secretions, feeding intolerance, or respiratory difficulties at birth should raise concern for EA. Failure to pass an orogastric tube into the stomach and the presence of abdominal bowel gas on plain film radiography suggests an EA with distal TEF (Gross type C, **Fig. 1**A). This is the most common form of EA/TEF and is found in about 85% of cases. Because the lower esophagus reaches the trachea, the gap between the esophageal segments is usually short.

An increased urgency for surgical repair exists in patients with EA with distal TEF because of the high risk of aspiration pneumonitis. If mechanical ventilation is required, gastric distention can further respiratory embarrassment. For this reason, positive pressure ventilation should be avoided whenever possible. Full aspiration precautions, including a Repogle-type orogastric tube to suction within the esophageal pouch, head of bed at 45°, and acid suppressive therapy, are initiated before operation. All neonates with EA/TEF should undergo a preoperative diagnostic workup looking for VACTERL anomalies. The most important component in this evaluation is the echocardiogram, because up to 35% will have cardiac abnormalities. The echocardiogram will also determine the side of the aortic arch, whether left or right. The most common operative approach for the repair of short-gap EA is a right thoracotomy because the aortic arch is on the left side in 95% of cases.[1,18] Through a muscle-sparing posterolateral incision, the fourth interspace is entered. Many surgeons advocate an extrapleural approach to minimize the risk of empyema and mediastinal sepsis should a postoperative esophageal leak occur.

In neonates with an EA and distal TEF, the goals of operative therapy are twofold: (1) to divide and close the fistula between the trachea and lower esophagus, and (2) to establish continuity of the esophagus. In most cases, the two ends of the esophagus are in proximity to each other, and a single-layer primary esophageal anastomosis can be performed. Postoperatively, the child returns to the intensive care unit with a chest tube in place and is weaned off of the ventilator. Feedings can be initiated through a transanastomotic tube 2 to 3 days after the operation in most cases. Seven days after the procedure, an esophagram is performed to check the integrity of the anastomosis. A leak is seen in approximately 15% of cases.[1,19] If no leak or significant stricture is identified, oral feedings are started, and the chest tube is removed. In the presence of a leak, continued parenteral nutrition, broad-spectrum antibiotics, and chest tube drainage will eventually allow the leak to close spontaneously in most cases.

Although many EA/TEF infants will have gastroesophageal reflux (GERD) after repair, only 15% to 20% will typically have severe and persistent symptoms that require an antireflux procedure, such as a Nissen fundoplication. Significant postoperative strictures are also not uncommon, but, if they occur, can be managed with serial endoscopic dilation.

Thoracoscopic Repair for Short-Gap Atresia

Pediatric thoracotomy incisions, even when muscle-sparing approaches are used, have been associated with several long-term complications, including shoulder weakness, winged scapula, and thoracic scoliosis.[20,21] Because of these morbidities and additional concerns regarding postoperative pain and cosmesis after thoracotomy, interest in neonatal thoracoscopic repair for short-gap EA has been increasing among pediatric surgeons. The procedure was first described in the late 1990s.[22–24] Proponents of thoracoscopic repair of EA/TEF have also touted the superior visualization provided by thoracoscopy compared with open surgery. Based on a recent United Kingdom–based survey of 100 pediatric surgeons, approximately 20% have successfully performed a repair of an EA/TEF using this minimally invasive approach.[25]

Because of the restricted working space of the neonatal thorax combined with the inherent difficulties of using thoracoscopic instruments to perform an esophageal anastomosis under tension, minimally invasive repair is a technically demanding procedure.[26] Consequently, the preferred candidates for thoracoscopic repair at the University of Michigan include those who have EA with distal TEF, are more than 2.5 kg in size, and have minimal cardiopulmonary disease. As in the open approach, close communication and cooperation among the entire operating room team remains essential for successful perioperative outcomes.

After the induction of general anesthesia, the airway is carefully assessed with rigid bronchoscopy to characterize the distal fistula and rule out a second, more proximal fistula. If the distal fistula is at or cephalad to the carina, a short-gap EA is confirmed. The child is then repositioned in a 30° or 45° prone decubitus position with the right chest up. Three or four ports are placed, and the right lung is collapsed with carbon dioxide insufflation to 4 to 8 mm Hg.

Except for the transpleural approach to the mediastinum, the thoracoscopic operation is conducted similarly to a standard thoracotomy repair. After the azygous vein is ligated, the distal esophagus is identified (**Fig. 2**A) and ligated at its entry into the trachea. The esophageal ends are mobilized, and an esophageal anastomosis is performed using multiple interrupted sutures (see **Fig. 2**B). Either intracorporeal or extracorporeal knot-tying techniques can be used. Before completion of the esophageal anastomosis, an 8-Fr transanastomotic feeding tube is advanced into the stomach. A chest tube is placed through one of the port sites and subsequently removed if no leak is documented on esophagram 7 days after repair.

In numerous reports of thoracoscopic EA/TEF repair, including a multicenter international series with 103 infants and a single institution series of 51 infants, clinical outcomes and postoperative complication rates have been reported to be comparable to those after traditional thoracotomy.[27–29] Approximately 30% require one or more endoscopic dilations of the anastomotic site. Unfortunately, operative times during thoracoscopic

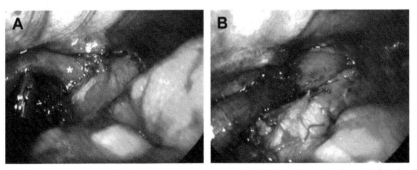

Fig. 2. Thoracoscopic repair of esophageal atresia with distal tracheoesophageal fistula. (*A*) Mobilization of the distal esophagus (*asterisk*) adjacent to the trachea. (*B*) Completed esophageal anastomosis.

repair tend to be longer, particularly during the learning phase of the procedure, and conversion rates to an open thoracotomy of up to 32% have been reported.[30]

LONG-GAP ATRESIA
Initial Management

When an orogastric tube cannot be passed into the stomach of a neonate found to have a gasless abdomen on the initial plain film, a long-gap atresia (defined as more than three vertebral bodies) should be suspected. The most common form of long-gap atresia is an isolated EA without a fistula to the airway (Gross type A, **Fig. 1**B). Although only 8% of children within the EA/TEF spectrum will have this variant, this is the second most common form of EA. Neonates with an isolated EA are at lower risk of aspiration pneumonitis than those with EA and a distal TEF. Nevertheless, isolated EA infants are more challenging to repair because of the long gap between the proximal and distal ends of the esophagus. Early primary repair of the esophagus in children with an isolated EA is usually not possible.[31]

The initial management of infants with an isolated EA includes screening for VACTERL anomalies and placement of a gastrostomy tube to allow feeding and evaluation of the lower esophagus. Historically, a cervical esophagostomy was advocated for long-gap EA, but this is no longer recommended because it will only make subsequent attempts at a primary esophageal repair more difficult.

The next procedure performed in isolated EA infants is an unstressed gapogram, a study that involves injecting radio-opaque contrast into the lower segment while a catheter is placed into the upper pouch. Alternatively, a neonatal endoscope can be used to help define the length of the lower esophageal segment on a gapogram study, but gentle pressure must be applied on the delicate newborn tissues to avoid distorting the true gap length. The authors' preference has been to use vertebral bodies as a unit of distance of the esophageal gap, because centimeters do not account for the different sizes of infants over time.[32]

The spectrum of gap lengths is wide because of considerable variation in the length of the lower esophagus, which can range from a tiny primordium to a longer segment reaching half way up the mediastinum. Accordingly, the appropriate method of repair may range from a primary repair under tension for shorter gaps to esophageal growth induction (Foker process) or conduit reconstruction for longer gaps. In the former situation, a delayed primary repair without any specific intervention in 1 to 3 months' time is possible because of spontaneous growth of the esophagus from swallowing attempts (proximal) and gastric reflux (distal).[33] A technique of delayed primary repair for up to 9 months using a modified Collis-Nissen procedure has also been reported.[34] At least one study has shown that selected infants can be managed safely at home on continuous upper pouch suction for months before definitive repair.[35]

Occasionally, an infant with EA with distal TEF may unexpectedly have a long gap identified intraoperatively. In this circumstance, maneuvers, including intra-abdominal esophageal mobilization and esophageal myotomy have been used to allow a primary repair. Although these maneuvers have been advocated to establish continuity, the authors generally discourage them, because they can also be associated with significant long-term problems, including strictures and GERD. In many cases, a delayed primary repair is a better option.

Conduit Reconstruction

In ultra-long-gap EA (defined as five or more vertebral bodies), a delayed primary repair after a trial of observation is usually not possible. One option for definitive reconstruction in these children is esophageal replacement with an autologous inter-position graft derived from stomach, colon, or jejunum.[3,19,36] These operations, which continue to remain in vogue at many referral centers worldwide, have been used successfully by pediatric surgeons for decades.[25,31,32,37]

The current debate in esophageal replacement surgery for long-gap EA continues to revolve around the best operation (eg, gastric transposition vs colon interposition), the benefits of minimally invasive techniques, and the appropriate timing of definitive reconstruction.[25] At the University of Michigan, among other institutions, gastric trans-position remains the preferred operation in most cases of ultra-long-gap EA.[31,32] The procedure requires only one anastomosis and can be performed via cervical and lapa-rotomy incisions, thereby entirely avoiding the morbidity of a thoracotomy. A minimally invasive approach has also been recently described.[37] A feeding jejunostomy placed during the procedure can help facilitate enteral nutrition postoperatively. Long-term concerns with gastric transposition include poor weight gain, anemia, pulmonary problems, reflux, and atrophic gastritis.

As with other technically challenging operations, surgeon experience with conduit reconstruction plays a major role in clinical outcomes. Because conduit construction is now uncommonly performed at most pediatric hospitals, referral of these cases to regional centers with expertise in these operative techniques is advised. Some pedi-atric surgeons have advocated for early esophageal replacement after a short trial of observation because it avoids the need for repeat operations and can be done with low morbidity and mortality when performed at an experienced center.[32,38] However, one should avoid abandoning the native esophagus too early, because a delayed primary repair may be possible in some of these children with long-gap EA.

Esophageal Growth Induction (Foker Process)

For more than a decade, the senior author (JEF) has been a champion of an alternative method for long-gap EA reconstruction based on the principle of continuous external traction on the esophagus.[39] This procedure, often referred to as the Foker process, is an inherently appealing approach to esophageal reconstruction because it induces esophageal growth and preserves the native esophagus, thereby enabling a true primary repair.[40] Esophageal growth induction has been shown to reliably increase the length and width of the esophagus, even when the lower esophagus begins as a very tiny primordium below the level of the diaphragm at birth (**Fig. 3**).[39,41]

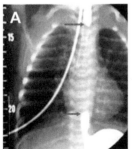 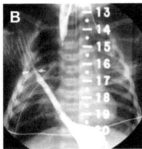 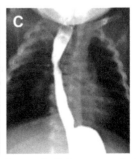

Fig. 3. Serial esophagrams after tension-induced esophageal growth (Foker process). (A) Preoperative esophagram with a high upper-esophageal segment and a lower segment that reached just above the diaphragm (arrows). (B) Esophageal segments on traction. The esophageal segments appear narrow, both from tension and because the contrast is not injected under pressure. (C) Postrepair study showing successful primary repair with anastomotic narrowing (arrow) that was subsequently treated with dilations.

Tension-induced esophageal growth has generated considerable interest within the pediatric surgical community because it represents a systematic, reproducible, and flexible approach to lengthen the esophagus. Among 84 pediatric surgeons in a recent survey, 33 (39%) preferred esophageal growth induction to other methods, including conduit reconstruction, for the management of long-gap EA.[25]

Although the application of tension to the esophagus is not an entirely new concept, many of the previously described strategies for lengthening the esophagus, including hydrostatic pressure, serial bougienage, magnets, internal traction, among others,[42–44] have never gained widespread popularity because of unreliable esophageal growth or high complication rates. The problems associated with these procedures are likely caused by a reliance on intermittent tension and growth induction of only the proximal or distal ends of the atretic esophagus.

The authors currently perform esophageal growth induction through a limited posterolateral thoracotomy incision. Thoracoscopic approaches have also been described.[39,45] Once adequate exposure is obtained, the proximal and distal esophagus are mobilized as much as possible. A very short distal esophagus near the diaphragm may require a second thoracotomy through the same skin incision to achieve complete distal mobilization. Four pledgeted horizontal mattress sutures (eg, 5-0 polypropylene) are placed through the esophageal wall adjacent to each of the atretic ends, being careful not enter the esophageal lumen (**Fig. 4**A). The sutures are tied and marked with clips adjacent to the atretic ends of the esophagus to enable subsequent assessment of the gap length on daily radiographs. Once all of the sutures are placed, they are externalized through the posterior chest wall in a crossed fashion and passed through silastic buttons before being tied under tension (see **Fig. 4**B).

Postoperatively, these children are kept in a position that minimizes trauma to the traction sutures. As esophageal growth occurs, tension is reestablished daily through the insertion of small pieces of silicone tubing under the traction sutures. Occasionally, the traction sutures can pull out of the esophagus, but the risks of salivary leak and mediastinitis remain low if the stitches have not entered the lumen (see **Fig. 4**A). Once the gap is less than two vertebral bodies in length, as shown by anterior and lateral chest radiographs, the patient undergoes another thoracotomy with primary repair of the esophagus.

Based on a literature review, the Foker process, or its various modifications as described by others, has been successfully used in more than 100 infants with long-gap EA at numerous centers worldwide.[39,46–51] As with all major operations, failures and complications have been reported after the procedure,[31] but the authors believe that most of these can be attributed to the learning curve and lack of familiarity with the many technical nuances required for consistent success. The largest experience to date with esophageal growth induction has been at the University of Minnesota and, more recently, Children's Hospital Boston, with excellent clinical results.[39]

In the senior author's personal case series, the procedure has enabled primary repair of the esophagus in all cases within 3 to 31 days (mean 14 ± 7 days, **Fig. 5**). As expected, longer time periods have been required in patients with the longest gaps and in those whose traction sutures pulled out with subsequent need for replacement. Serial radiographs have shown the gap closing at an average rate of 0.53 ± 0.2 cm per day. The rates have been higher initially because of the contribution of stretch, and decrease to 0.2 ± 0.1 cm per day later in the growth period. With the upper measurement boundary of the fifth cervical vertebrae, the preoperative length of the upper pouch has ranged from 0.2 to 5.4 cm (2.5 ± 1.2

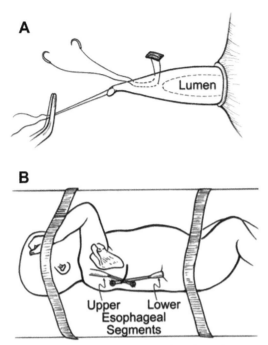

Fig. 4. Esophageal growth induction. (*A*) Placement of pledgeted traction sutures. Deep bites into the segment are taken, with care not to enter the lumen. Four sutures are typically placed on each segment. (*B*) External traction configuration during the procedure. The sutures are brought out posteriorly on the chest wall. The upper segment sutures exit above the thoracotomy incision while the lower segment sutures are brought out below. Traction is placed on the segments by threading the sutures through silastic buttons on the skin surface. Small pieces of silastic tubing are placed under the sutures to increase the tension. (*From* Foker JE, Kendall TC, Catton K, et al. A flexible approach to achieve a true primary repair for all infants with esophageal atresia. Semin Pediatr Surg 2005;14(1):11–2; with permission.)

cm) and has grown to 3.4 to 8.4 cm (5.5 ± 1.3 cm), a percentage increase of 16% to 1702% (mean, 197%). Preoperatively, the lower esophagus was often small and ranged from 0.2 to 3.2 cm (1.8 ± 0.8 cm, **Fig. 5**). The length after growth has ranged from 1.9 to 9.2 cm (4.7 ± 1.3 cm) with a percent increase range of 59% to 2350%

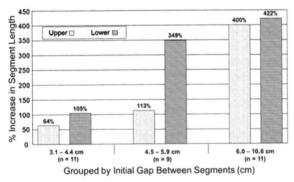

Fig. 5. Tension-induced growth of the upper and lower esophageal segments, grouped by initial gap length.

(mean, 288%). In 16% of patients, poor growth rates necessitated another thoracotomy to either reconfigure or replace traction sutures that had pulled out.[52]

When the results of tension-induced esophageal growth were first reported, critics of the procedure argued that the esophagus was merely being stretched under continuous axial tension over time. Both experimental and human data do not support this contention. In a rat animal model of EA, continuous traction on the esophagus has been shown to increase esophageal mass without major tissue damage.[53] Moreover, high-resolution endoscopic ultrasound wall measurements in infants undergoing the Foker process further support the notion of true esophageal growth. For example, in a recent study of 11 patients, esophageal wall thickness (2 mm) was similar before growth stimulation and after esophageal anastomosis, suggesting that the walls did not become attenuated by increased tension.[54] The muscularis propria was 0.8 ± 0.2 mm, the mucosa and submucosa together were 1.0 ± 0.2 mm, and the serosa layer was 0.2 ± 0.04 mm.

The overall functional results in patients having undergone esophageal growth induction with eventual primary repair are of obvious importance.[55] As expected, anastomotic strictures are common but are usually amendable to endoscopic dilation. A small number of infants with resistant strictures have required segmental resection. Unfortunately, severe GERD and reflux esophagitis have been the norm in this patient population despite the fact that the gastroesophageal junction remains below the diaphragm, and more than 95% have eventually required a Nissen fundoplication.[55] Of the 42 patients who were at least 3 years beyond primary repair after this procedure, all but one has been able to eat a normal oral diet for age. Only those with significant syndromes have required a gastrostomy tube. Ongoing and concurrent multidisciplinary collaboration between pediatric surgeons, gastroenterologists, and feeding specialists remains paramount to optimize clinical outcomes. No comparative studies of esophageal growth induction with other methods of esophageal reconstruction have been performed in patients with long-gap EA.

SUMMARY

The diagnosis and treatment of patients along the EA/TEF spectrum continues to evolve within the field of pediatric surgery. Despite refinements in fetal imaging, prenatal diagnosis remains difficult. Most patients with short-gap EA are now candidates for thoracoscopic repair, which offers the promise of lower surgical morbidity when performed by advanced minimally invasive surgeons. Large comparative studies remain sparse but suggest equivalent outcomes compared with open thoracotomy. As the technology associated with minimally invasive surgery continues to improve, the authors believe that it is only a matter of time until more of these repairs are conducted without thoracotomy.

Regarding infants with long-gap EA, tension-induced growth of the esophagus now serves as a viable alternative to conduit reconstruction, including gastric transposition. In centers that have significant experience with esophageal growth induction, successful primary repair of the esophagus has been possible in most cases. Although the precise role of tension-induced growth relative to conduit reconstruction remains one of ongoing debate, it is difficult to argue against the flexibility of former procedure and the inherent advantages of a primary esophageal repair, which has been a central tenet of esophageal surgery for more than 60 years. Further accumulation of long-term data in patients undergoing esophageal growth induction should help clarify appropriate patient selection and enable more objective comparisons of outcomes after the different operations.

REFERENCES

1. Manning PB, Morgan RA, Coran AG, et al. Fifty years' experience with esophageal atresia and tracheoesophageal fistula. Beginning with Cameron Haight's first operation in 1935. Ann Surg 1986;204(4):446–53.
2. Haight C. Congenital atresia of the esophagus with tracheoesophageal fistula: reconstruction of esophageal continuity by primary anastomosis. Ann Surg 1944;120(4):623–52.
3. Spitz L. Esophageal atresia. Lessons I have learned in a 40-year experience. J Pediatr Surg 2006;41(10):1635–40.
4. El-Gohary Y, Gittes GK, Tovar JA. Congenital anomalies of the esophagus. Semin Pediatr Surg 2010;19(3):186–93.
5. Shaw-Smith C. Oesophageal atresia, tracheo-oesophageal fistula, and the VACTERL association: review of genetics and epidemiology. J Med Genet 2006;43(7):545–54.
6. Quan L, Smith DW. The VATER association. Vertebral defects, Anal atresia, T-E fistula with esophageal atresia, Radial and Renal dysplasia: a spectrum of associated defects. J Pediatr 1973;82(1):104–7.
7. de Jong EM, de Haan MA, Gischler SJ, et al. Pre- and postnatal diagnosis and outcome of fetuses and neonates with esophageal atresia and tracheoesophageal fistula. Prenat Diagn 2010;30(3):274–9.
8. Houben CH, Curry JI. Current status of prenatal diagnosis, operative management and outcome of esophageal atresia/tracheo-esophageal fistula. Prenat Diagn 2008;28(7):667–75.
9. Sparey C, Jawaheer G, Barrett AM, et al. Esophageal atresia in the Northern Region Congenital Anomaly Survey, 1985-1997: prenatal diagnosis and outcome. Am J Obstet Gynecol 2000;182(2):427–31.
10. Brantberg A, Blaas HG, Haugen SE, et al. Esophageal obstruction-prenatal detection rate and outcome. Ultrasound Obstet Gynecol 2007;30(2):180–7.
11. Stringel G, Lawrence C, McBride W. Repair of long gap esophageal atresia without anastomosis. J Pediatr Surg 2010;45(5):872–5.
12. Houfflin-Debarge V, Bigot J. Ultrasound and MRI prenatal diagnosis of esophageal atresia: effect on management. J Pediatr Gastroenterol Nutr 2011;52(Suppl 1): S9–11.
13. Shulman A, Mazkereth R, Zalel Y, et al. Prenatal identification of esophageal atresia: the role of ultrasonography for evaluation of functional anatomy. Prenat Diagn 2002;22(8):669–74.
14. Has R, Gunay S. Upper neck pouch sign in prenatal diagnosis of esophageal atresia. Arch Gynecol Obstet 2004;270(1):56–8.
15. Langer JC, Hussain H, Khan A, et al. Prenatal diagnosis of esophageal atresia using sonography and magnetic resonance imaging. J Pediatr Surg 2001; 36(5):804–7.
16. Salomon LJ, Sonigo P, Ou P, et al. Real-time fetal magnetic resonance imaging for the dynamic visualization of the pouch in esophageal atresia. Ultrasound Obstet Gynecol 2009;34(4):471–4.
17. Czerkiewicz I, Dreux S, Beckmezian A, et al. Biochemical amniotic fluid pattern for prenatal diagnosis of esophageal atresia. Pediatr Res 2011;70(2):199–202.
18. Mortell AE, Azizkhan RG. Esophageal atresia repair with thoracotomy: the Cincinnati contemporary experience. Semin Pediatr Surg 2009;18(1):12–9.
19. Tsai JY, Berkery L, Wesson DE, et al. Esophageal atresia and tracheoesophageal fistula: surgical experience over two decades. Ann Thorac Surg 1997;64(3): 778–83 [discussion: 783–4].

20. Jaureguizar E, Vazquez J, Murcia J, et al. Morbid musculoskeletal sequelae of thoracotomy for tracheoesophageal fistula. J Pediatr Surg 1985;20(5):511–4.
21. Lawal TA, Gosemann JH, Kuebler JF, et al. Thoracoscopy versus thoracotomy improves midterm musculoskeletal status and cosmesis in infants and children. Ann Thorac Surg 2009;87(1):224–8.
22. Rothenberg SS. Thoracoscopic repair of tracheoesophageal fistula in newborns. J Pediatr Surg 2002;37(6):869–72.
23. Bax KM, van Der Zee DC. Feasibility of thoracoscopic repair of esophageal atresia with distal fistula. J Pediatr Surg 2002;37(2):192–6.
24. van der Zee DC, Bax NM. Thoracoscopic repair of esophageal atresia with distal fistula. Surg Endosc 2003;17(7):1065–7.
25. Ron O, De Coppi P, Pierro A. The surgical approach to esophageal atresia repair and the management of long-gap atresia: results of a survey. Semin Pediatr Surg 2009;18(1):44–9.
26. Rothenberg SS. Thoracoscopic repair of esophageal atresia and tracheo-esophageal fistula in neonates: evolution of a technique. J Laparoendosc Adv Surg Tech A 2012;22(2):195–9.
27. Holcomb GW 3rd, Rothenberg SS, Bax KM, et al. Thoracoscopic repair of esophageal atresia and tracheoesophageal fistula: a multi-institutional analysis. Ann Surg 2005;242(3):422–8 [discussion: 428–30].
28. Lugo B, Malhotra A, Guner Y, et al. Thoracoscopic versus open repair of tracheoesophageal fistula and esophageal atresia. J Laparoendosc Adv Surg Tech A 2008;18(5):753–6.
29. van der Zee DC, Bax KN. Thoracoscopic treatment of esophageal atresia with distal fistula and of tracheomalacia. Semin Pediatr Surg 2007;16(4):224–30.
30. Szavay PO, Zundel S, Blumenstock G, et al. Perioperative outcome of patients with esophageal atresia and tracheo-esophageal fistula undergoing open versus thoracoscopic surgery. J Laparoendosc Adv Surg Tech A 2011;21(5):439–43.
31. Holland AJ, Ron O, Pierro A, et al. Surgical outcomes of esophageal atresia without fistula for 24 years at a single institution. J Pediatr Surg 2009;44(10):1928–32.
32. Cowles RA, Coran AG. Gastric transposition in infants and children. Pediatr Surg Int 2010;26(12):1129–34.
33. Puri P, Khurana S. Delayed primary esophageal anastomosis for pure esophageal atresia. Semin Pediatr Surg 1998;7(2):126–9.
34. Nakahara Y, Aoyama K, Goto T, et al. Modified Collis-Nissen procedure for long gap pure esophageal atresia. J Pediatr Surg 2012;47(3):462–6.
35. Aziz D, Schiller D, Gerstle JT, et al. Can 'long-gap' esophageal atresia be safely managed at home while awaiting anastomosis? J Pediatr Surg 2003;38(5):705–8.
36. Hirschl RB, Yardeni D, Oldham K, et al. Gastric transposition for esophageal replacement in children: experience with 41 consecutive cases with special emphasis on esophageal atresia. Ann Surg 2002;236(4):531–9 [discussion: 539–41].
37. St Peter SD, Ostlie DJ. Laparoscopic gastric transposition with cervical esophagogastric anastomosis for long gap pure esophageal atresia. J Laparoendosc Adv Surg Tech A 2010;20(1):103–6.
38. Sharma S, Gupta DK. Primary gastric pull-up in pure esophageal atresia: technique, feasibility and outcome. A prospective observational study. Pediatr Surg Int 2011;27(6):583–5.
39. Foker JE, Kendall TC, Catton K, et al. A flexible approach to achieve a true primary repair for all infants with esophageal atresia. Semin Pediatr Surg 2005;14(1):8–15.

40. Foker JE, Linden BC, Boyle EM Jr, et al. Development of a true primary repair for the full spectrum of esophageal atresia. Ann Surg 1997;226(4):533–41 [discussion: 541–3].
41. Till H, Rolle U, Siekmeyer W, et al. Combination of spit fistula advancement and external traction for primary repair of long-gap esophageal atresia. Ann Thorac Surg 2008;86(6):1969–71.
42. Kimura K, Soper RT. Multistaged extrathoracic esophageal elongation for long gap esophageal atresia. J Pediatr Surg 1994;29(4):566–8.
43. Vogel AM, Yang EY, Fishman SJ. Hydrostatic stretch-induced growth facilitating primary anastomosis in long-gap esophageal atresia. J Pediatr Surg 2006; 41(6):1170–2.
44. Hendren WH, Hale JR. Electromagnetic bougienage to lengthen esophageal segments in congenital esophageal atresia. N Engl J Med 1975;293(9):428–32.
45. van der Zee DC, Vieirra-Travassos D, Kramer WL, et al. Thoracoscopic elongation of the esophagus in long gap esophageal atresia. J Pediatr Surg 2007;42(10): 1785–8.
46. Al-Qahtani AR, Yazbeck S, Rosen NG, et al. Lengthening technique for long gap esophageal atresia and early anastomosis. J Pediatr Surg 2003;38(5):737–9.
47. Till H, Muensterer OJ, Rolle U, et al. Staged esophageal lengthening with internal and subsequent external traction sutures leads to primary repair of an ultralong gap esophageal atresia with upper pouch tracheoesophagel fistula. J Pediatr Surg 2008;43(6):E33–5.
48. Skarsgard ED. Dynamic esophageal lengthening for long gap esophageal atresia: experience with two cases. J Pediatr Surg 2004;39(11):1712–4.
49. Hadidi AT, Hosie S, Waag KL. Long gap esophageal atresia: lengthening technique and primary anastomosis. J Pediatr Surg 2007;42(10):1659–62.
50. Lopes MF, Reis A, Coutinho S, et al. Very long gap esophageal atresia successfully treated by esophageal lengthening using external traction sutures. J Pediatr Surg 2004;39(8):1286–7.
51. Gaglione G, Tramontano A, Capobianco A, et al. Foker's technique in oesophageal atresia with double fistula: a case report. Eur J Pediatr Surg 2003;13(1): 50–3.
52. Khan KM, Sabati AA, Kendall T, et al. The effect of traction on esophageal structure in children with long-gap esophageal atresia. Dig Dis Sci 2006;51(11): 1917–21.
53. Lopes MF, Catre D, Cabrita A, et al. Effect of traction sutures in the distal esophagus of the rat: a model for esophageal elongation by Foker's method. Dis Esophagus 2008;21(6):570–3.
54. Khan KM, Foker JE. Use of high-resolution endoscopic ultrasonography to examine the effect of tension on the esophagus during primary repair of long-gap esophageal atresia. Pediatr Radiol 2007;37(1):41–5.
55. Khan KM, Krosch TC, Eickhoff JC, et al. Achievement of feeding milestones after primary repair of long-gap esophageal atresia. Early Hum Dev 2009;85(6): 387–92.

Innovations in the Surgical Management of Congenital Diaphragmatic Hernia

KuoJen Tsao, MD[a,b,c,]*, Kevin P. Lally, MD, MS[a,c]

KEYWORDS

- Congenital diaphragmatic hernia • Minimally invasive surgery • Tissue engineering
- Diaphragmatic patch

KEY POINTS

- The mortality for neonatal congenital diaphragmatic hernia has not improved in the last 15-25 years. Despite improved understandings in the pathophysiology, the overall survival is approximately 68%.
- Recent advances in neonatal congenital diaphragmatic hernia have focused on surgical approaches and diaphragmatic replacements. Both have attempted to reduce the morbidity associated with surgical repair of CDH.
- Better understanding of clinical outcomes requires a risk-stratified approach to analysis. This is dependent on a standardized classification of risk and disease severity.

OBJECTIVES

- Understand the surgical approaches to the repair of congenital diaphragmatic hernia as well as their associated morbidity.
- Understand the current options for diaphragmatic replacement.

INTRODUCTION

Congenital diaphragmatic hernia (CDH) remains one of the most challenging neonatal diseases for pediatric surgeons and neonatologists. The spectrum of disease can range from asymptomatic, undiagnosed defects that present later in life to those with immediate respiratory distress that result in neonatal death. Despite the overwhelming interest and research in CDH, there has been minimal improvement in outcomes in the last 15 to 25 years since the adoption of delayed surgical repair with permissive hypercapnea and gentle ventilation.[1]

Financial disclosures: None.
[a] Department of Pediatric Surgery, The University of Texas School of Medicine at Houston, Houston, TX, USA; [b] Department of Surgery, The University of Texas School of Medicine at Houston, Houston, TX, USA; [c] The Children's Memorial Hermann Hospital, Houston, TX, USA
* Department of Pediatric Surgery, The University of Texas School of Medicine at Houston, 6431 Fannin Street, Suite 5.254, Houston, TX 77030.
E-mail address: kuojen.tsao@uth.tmc.edu

Until the late 1980s the overall survival rate was approximately 50%,[2,3] with rates individual centers ranging between 20% and 70%.[1,4] Today, survival has improved with a reported overall rate of 68%,[5] while innovative therapies such as perfluorocarbon-induced lung growth[6] and fetal tracheal occlusion[7,8] continue to be evaluated. Innovations in the surgical treatment of CDH have focused on reduction in morbidity, specifically on surgical approaches and alternative diaphragmatic replacements. In addition, understanding the need for risk-adjustment analysis in rare diseases has enhanced the interpretation of clinical outcomes.

SURGICAL APPROACH
Minimally Invasive Techniques

The surgical repair of CDH has been traditionally performed via an open thoracic or abdominal approach. Laparotomy provides several advantages over thoracotomy, including easier reduction of intrathoracic viscera, ability to mobilize the posterior rim of diaphragm, easier management of intestinal rotational anomalies, and avoidance of thoracotomy-associated musculoskeletal sequelae. The vast majority of neonatal repairs for CDH are through a subcostal laparotomy (91%).[9]

However, the morbidity and respiratory sequelae of open repair of CDH remains a concern. In addition to the CDH-related effects of pulmonary hypoplasia and hypertension, reduction in abdominal and chest wall compliance after repair may exacerbate the pathophysiology of severe CDH. In hopes of minimizing the postoperative effects, surgeons have increasingly adopted a minimally invasive surgery (MIS) approached to the repair of CDH since Silen reported the first MIS repair of an adolescent Bochdalek-type CDH in 1995.[10] Data from the Congenital Diaphragmatic Hernia Registry demonstrate that operative techniques include open abdominal and thoracic approaches as well as laparoscopic and thoracoscopic strategies, and that MIS techniques have been used in 20 of the 93 centers (21.5%).[11] Comparative evidence between MIS and open approaches has been limited to single-institution experiences or retrospective analysis.[11–17] Proponents of MIS tout benefits in cosmesis with smaller incisions, decreased postoperative pain, and possible improvements in postoperative pulmonary compliance, while minimizing complications of thoracotomy and laparotomy such as incisional hernias, chest wall deformities, musculoskeletal maladies, and adhesive intestinal obstruction.

The sensitivity of CDH infants to hypercapnea and acidosis has drawn concerns regarding the utilization of MIS, for 2 major reasons: (1) CDH neonates may absorb the CO_2 used for insufflation[18,19] and (2) insufflation with CO_2 may raise intracavity pressures thus limiting venous return, end-organ perfusion, and tidal volume. The combination of CDH-related pulmonary hypoplasia, pulmonary hypertension, and labile pulmonary vascular reactivity may compromise physiology in the operating room. Although increases in CO_2 absorption during MIS are generally well tolerated in infants, CDH neonates specifically demonstrate greater changes in end-tidal CO_2 ($Etco_2$) and impaired elimination of CO_2 during thoracoscopy and laparoscopy.[20,21] Hypercapnea and the associated acidosis may result in increased pulmonary shunting. Because of these concerns, the selection criteria for infants undergoing MIS repairs should be carefully scrutinized. Centers that perform thoracoscopic CDH repairs have advocated for stringent intraoperative monitoring of $Etco_2$ and arterial partial pressure of CO_2.[22]

With increased surgeon experience and improved understanding of the physiology of MIS and CDH repair, selection criteria for patients have also expanded. Historically, MIS approaches were reserved for stable infants with anticipated small defects. Using anatomic markers such as stomach herniation, surgeons have attempted to predict which defects are amenable to MIS repairs.[23] Initially the presence of the nasogastric tube within the abdomen on radiograph, suggesting an intact esophageal hiatus with stomach and liver in the abdomen as well as minimal respiratory compromise (peak inspiratory pressures [PIP] <24 mm Hg), were thought to be associated with success-ful thoracoscopic repair. Gourlay and colleagues[24] reported 95% success rates with thoracoscopic repair when patients demonstrated absence of significant congenital cardiac anomaly, absence of preoperative extracorporeal membrane oxygenation therapy (ECMO), PIP 26 cm H_2O or less, and Oxygenation Index 5 or less on the day of surgery. Today, the application of MIS has expanded to those infants with more severe sequelae of CDH. For example, infants requiring preoperative ECMO have undergone successful repair with a MIS approach.[18,25] In addition, large defects that require patch repairs[18,24,26] and right-sided defects are no longer contraindica-tions to MIS.[27]

Despite demonstration of the ability to perform the repair via an MIS approach, little assessment of short-term and long-term outcomes regarding the durability and recur-rence rates for MIS techniques has been performed. Early recurrence rates have been reported to be as high as 23% to 33% from individual centers,[13,15] while the recur-rence rate for thoracoscopic repairs was 16.1% compared with 4.9% for open repairs in one study (relative risk 3.21; 95% confidence interval [CI] 1.11–9.29). In a recent review of the CDH Registry, MIS repairs were performed in only 3.4% infants with CDH, with a significantly higher in-hospital recurrence rate for MIS repairs (7.9% vs 2.7%, P<.05). Thoracoscopic CDH repairs had the highest rate of recurrence, at 8.8%. The odds ratio (OR) for recurrence with MIS was 3.59 (95% CI 1.92–6.71) after adjusting for gestational age, birth weight, patch repair, and need for ECMO. A meta-analysis of neonatal MIS repair for CDH identified only 3 relevant studies with a total of 143 patients.[16] Thus, the current evidence is subject to the pitfalls of retrospective studies, that is, selection bias and inadequate follow-up, and our understanding of long-term outcomes remains limited.

Robotic Techniques

Robotic repair of congenital diaphragmatic anomalies have been demonstrated to be feasible and safe.[28–30] Advances in 5-mm robotic instrumentation in the last 10 years have allowed operative access to neonatal patients. Proponents of robotic CDH repair tout the increased degrees of freedom of the articulating instruments for suturing. Bochdalek-type and Morgagni-type hernias have been repaired with robotic assis-tance via a laparoscopic or thoracoscopic approach.[30] Slater and Meehan[30] reported their experience with robotic repairs of diaphragmatic anomalies in 8 patients with an average weight of 3.6 kg (range 2.2–10.5 kg) including 5 patients with Bochdalek-type hernias. Two patients required conversion to conventional MIS techniques and one patient developed a recurrence, with an average follow-up of 18 months. Although the thoracic approach was preferred, the surgeons suggested that an abdominal approach may be better for smaller newborns less than 2.5 kg because of the increased space required for the articulating instruments. Although the long-term outcomes remain unclear, continued improvements in technology provide promise for robotic surgery for CDH.

DIAPHRAGMATIC REPLACEMENTS

Repair of large diaphragmatic hernias is a surgical challenge for pediatric surgeons. According the CDH Registry, 48.3% of infants undergoing repair require a patch.[31] When primary repair is not possible, diaphragmatic replacement with a prosthetic patch or autologous tissue becomes necessary. Comparative studies between patch and no-patch repairs have consistently shown increased morbidity and mortality in the patch groups, most likely due to the underlying defect size and the associated severity of the pulmonary hypoplasia.[32,33] In many clinical research studies, patch repair is used as a surrogate for defect size and disease severity (ie, larger defect leads to increased severity of respiratory disease).[11,31]

The options for patches consisting of nonabsorbable synthetic or absorbable biosynthetic materials have increased over the last 20 years (**Box 1**).

Nonabsorbable Synthetic Patches

Nonbiodegradable materials such as polytetrafluoroethylene (PTFE or Gore-Tex) or composite-mesh polypropylene (Marlex) are routinely used to provide a tension-free repair of CDH.[9] Synthetic patches are commonly used for several reasons: (1) they are easily sized to fit the diaphragmatic defect, (2) less tissue dissection and mobilization is required, thus reducing the risk of hemorrhage when repair is performed on ECMO, and (3) they can be used immediately and require minimal preparation time. Synthetic patches represent the majority of the mesh diaphragmatic replacements used in neonates with large CDH.[34]

There are several disadvantages to synthetic patches for the repair of CDH. The overall recurrence rate has been reported to be as high as 50%.[34] Recurrence with PTFE appears to be bimodal, with an early peak in the first months after repair and late recurrences years later.[34] Early recurrences are most likely due to inadequate tissue adhesion or scarring, as may be seen with large defects with small or incomplete muscular rim that requires anchoring to the ribs or esophagus. PTFE tends to scar and shrink diaphragm over time, which may lead to late recurrences in the growing child. Several techniques have been described in an effort to prevent CDH recurrence. Loff and colleagues[35] constructed a cone-shaped, double-fixed PTFE

Box 1
Diaphragm replacements

Nonabsorbable synthetic patches

    Polytetrafluoroethylene (PTFE) (Gore-Tex)

    PTFE and polypropylene (Marlex)

Absorbable biosynthetic patches

    Porcine intestinal submucosa (Surgisis)

    Porcine dermal collagen (Permacol)

    Human cadaveric dermis (AlloDerm)

    Fetal bovine dermal collage (Surgimend)

    Polylactic-co-glycolic acid (PLGA)

Autologous tissue patches

    Reverse latissimus dorsi muscle

    Serratus anterior muscle

    Internal oblique/transversus abdominis muscles

Tissue-engineered patches

    Amniotic fluid, stem cell–derived muscle

patch to allow the patch to expand over time. As a result, the recurrence rate decreased from 46% to 9% in the first year after repair. Others have used a mesh plug and patch in the setting of recurrent CDH repair, with similar results.[36] Riehle and colleagues[37] described use of a double-sided composite patch consisting of PTFE on one side and type-1 monofilament, macroporous polypropylene (Marlex) on the other. Using a pledgeted, nonabsorbable running suture for fixation, recurrence occurred in 1 of 46 patients with a mean follow-up of 49 months.

Although prosthetic patches seem to be a good initial solution, long-term complications appear to be increased with nonabsorbable materials. Patches, such as PTFE, that are anchored to the chest wall can potentially produce a tethering point and may contribute to pectus-type deformities.[14,38] Other investigators have described an increased incidence of bowel obstruction, need for splenectomy, patch infections, and abdominal wall deformities.[34,39]

Absorbable Biosynthetic Patches

In efforts to avoid the aforementioned complications related to synthetic patches, alternatives to prosthetic materials have been introduced. Absorbable biosynthetic materials offer lower risks of infection and the ability to grow with the patient. Surgisis is an acellular, bioengineered porcine intestinal submucosal matrix that consists of a type-I collagen lattice with embedded growth factors. This non–cross-linked biological matrix is absorbed into the tissue bed, and promotes fibroblast migration and cellular differentiation.[40] First used to repair incisional, inguinal, and paraesophageal hernias,[41,42] Surgisis has been widely used for the repair of CDH.[10] Despite the demonstrated engraftment and neovascularization, recurrence rates for Surgisis appear to be similar when compared with Gore-Tex.[32] However, Surgisis demonstrated a higher rate of small bowel obstruction (31% for Surgisis vs 9% for Gore-Tex).

Permacol is an acellular sheet of porcine dermal collagen consisting of cross-linked lysine and hydroxylysine residues within the collagen fibers that promote a minimal inflammatory process. Theoretically, with inflammation similar to that of wound healing the neodiaphragm is more pliable and, subsequently, less prone to recurrence. In a study by Mitchell and colleagues,[43] there were no recurrences observed with Permacol in 8 patients with a median follow-up of 20 months, whereas recurrences were noted in 2% of patients with primary repair and 28% of diaphragms reconstructed with Gore-Tex.

Several other biosynthetic patches have been developed and used in the repair of CDH. AlloDerm is an acellular human cadaveric dermis that is cross-linked for rapid revascularization. This patch requires a 2-step rehydration process. Animal studies have demonstrated revascularization and cell repopulation within 1 month.[44] Surgimend is an acellular fetal bovine dermal collagen. Consisting of interwoven collagen, Surgimend may promote increased type-III collagen of fetal origin that contributes to scarless wound healing. Because there is no cross-linking there is an increased collagen resistance to collagenase, leading to greater durability. Polylactic-co-glycolic acid (PLGA) is a collagen scaffold that promotes neovascularization and autologous tissue regeneration. Animal studies have demonstrated ingrowth of fibroblasts, resulting in a thicker neodiaphragm.[45]

Despite the theoretical advantages, absorbable biosynthetic patches remain imperfect. Materials such as Surgisis have demonstrated thinning and incomplete muscular ingrowth.[46] Vascular ingrowth may be difficult, especially in large defects where native diaphragmatic muscle is absent. Albeit from different causes, biosynthetic patches are prone to recurrent hernia formation, much like nonabsorbable patches.[47] In addition, organ adherence, often to the small bowel, spleen, or liver, appears to be required for neovascularization.[39,48] Consequently, biological patches may also be associated with adhesive bowel obstruction.[32,39,47] Because of these many disadvantages, biosynthetic patches have fallen out of favor with many surgeons.[9]

Autologous Tissue Patches

Persistent complications with synthetic and biosynthetic patches have prompted some surgeons to advocate for primary repair with autologous muscle flaps, or staged reconstruction of large diaphragmatic defects with an initial synthetic patch followed by an autologous muscle flap.[14] Muscle flaps offer the advantage of using a vascularized tissue that will grow with the infant.

Several different abdominal muscle flaps have been described as a diaphragmatic replacement. In 1962, Meeker and Snyder[49] first described using anterior abdominal wall for repair of a CDH. In 1971, Simpson and Gossage[50] described use of a split abdominal wall muscle flap to repair a large defect in a 1-day-old neonate. Scaife and colleagues[51] described using a split abdominal muscle flap of the internal oblique and transversus abdominis muscles for primary repair of large diaphragmatic hernias. Using a lower abdominal incision the transversus abdominis was utilized to repair a CDH, with complete agenesis of the diaphragm on ECMO. This approach appears to have minimized the hemorrhagic risk while repairing a CDH on ECMO, owing to the avascular dissection plane between the muscle layers.[52]

Chest wall muscles have also been used to repair diaphragmatic hernia. The reverse latissimus dorsi muscle flap was first described by Bianchi and colleagues[53] in 1983. Based on the lumbar perforating blood vessels, the reverse latissimus dorsi muscle provides a wide pedicle for a tension-free repair. For very large defects, such as agenesis of the diaphragm, combined use of the latissimus dorsi and serratus anterior muscles has been described.[54–56] Although autologous muscle flaps are vascularized and tend to grow with the child, these diaphragmatic reconstructions with latissimus dorsi/serratus muscle flaps are typically small and have demonstrated atrophy over time because of denervation of the graft. In addition, the lack of innervation prevents the natural physiologic movement of the muscle flap. As a result, some surgeons have advocated using the reverse latissimus dorsi flap with a microneural anastomosis of the phrenic nerve to the thoracodorsal nerve, to prevent muscle atrophy and to allow physiologic muscle movement.[55,57] Sydorak and colleagues[55] described their initial experience with this technique in 7 infants with CDH. At a median age of 24 months, the investigators demonstrated fluoroscopic evidence of nonparadoxic neodiaphragmatic motion resulting from phrenic nerve innervation, including evidence of phrenic nerve conduction.

The disadvantage with using local muscle flaps is the associated deformity of the body wall.[58] Consequently, muscle flaps have been primarily reserved for reconstruction in the setting of recurrent CDH. Although the risk of infection is low and growth is observed with autologous tissue, recurrence is a risk, attributable to atrophy of a denervated muscle flap.[55]

Tissue-Engineered Patches

As may be seen from the foregoing discussion, the ideal diaphragmatic replacement remains elusive in the operative treatment of CDH. Advances in regenerative medicine may provide alternatives for diaphragmatic repair. For example, tissue-engineered muscle may provide a patch of functional skeletal muscle that may not atrophy and has minimal risk of infection. Although the supporting 3-dimensional scaffold is a key component of tissue engineering, skeletal muscle regeneration relies on a cell source with myogenic potential.[59,60] Amniotic fluid–derived stem cells may be a safe and abundant source of cells with myogenic potential.[61] Collected at the time of amniocentesis, amniotic stem cells could be used to engineer a muscular patch to be used during postnatal repair. Fuchs and colleagues[62] have developed a fetal tissue–based diaphragmatic construct by using autologous tendon engineered from mesenchymal amniocytes. Improved mechanical and functional outcomes offer promise for clinical application in the near future when compared with acellular bio-prosthetic patches in preclinical studies.[63]

RISK STRATIFICATION FOR CDH

Rare diseases, such as CDH, present major challenges in clinical care as well as in interpretation of clinical outcomes. Because of the wide spectrum of disease severity, most centers have highly variable experience in the severity of CDH from year to year with most advanced therapies.[64] As such, clinical evidence has been limited in quality and only to broad conclusions.[11,31]

The size of the diaphragmatic defect has been associated with severity of disease.[65,66] The Congenital Diaphragmatic Hernia Study Group (CDHSG) classified CDH based on the size of the defect and type of repair: primary repairs, repairs with patch that were not agenesis of the diaphragm, and agenesis of the diaphragm.[66] The overall mortality for patients with agenesis of the diaphragm was 43%, with an OR of 14.07 (95% CI 10.35–19.13) in comparison with primarily repaired defects. The association between defect size and disease severity has prompted development of a universal grading system that uses a diagrammatic schema to define CDH defect size. The 4 classifications range from small defects that could be repaired primarily to total diaphragmatic agenesis based on intraoperative findings (**Fig. 1**). Using other variables of comorbidity and disease

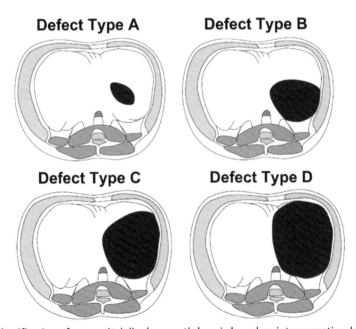

Fig. 1. Classification of congenital diaphragmatic hernia based on intraoperative defect size. Diagrams are drawn with the diaphragmatic defect on the patient's left from an abdominal approach. (*From* Tsao K, Lally KP. The Congenital Diaphragmatic Hernia Study Group: a voluntary international registry. Semin Pediatr Surg 2008;17:90–7. CDH website. Available at: http://utsurg.uth.tmc.edu/pedisurgery/cdhsg/index.html. Accessed April 13, 2012.)

severity, the CDHSG is attempting to provide an evidence-based risk-stratification classification of CDH. This issue is particularly prudent when innovative therapies are introduced, so as to ensure appropriate comparative analysis.

SUMMARY

Despite improvements in survival and major paradigm shifts in management, consensus treatment and management of infants with CDH remain elusive. Quality clinical evidence to support many modalities is limited. Most outcomes data are reported from either single-center experiences,[67–69] hospital databases,[70] or network registries.[71–73] There remain a limited number of prospective controlled clinical trials that examine various interventions for infants with CDH.[6,74–76] As such, the evidence to support innovations in surgical treatment of CDH suffers from low-quality clinical evidence, often attributable to compromises in study design and limitations of sample size. According to the CDH Registry, the average number of CDH infants seen per center is less than 10 per year.[64] Even high-volume centers may have limited experience with novel treatment modalities because of the broad spectrum of disease. Although many advances in the treatment of CDH demonstrate promise, outcomes data for novel CDH therapies should be carefully evaluated, with an understanding of risk stratification, before the adoption of any new treatment.

REFERENCES

1. Boloker J, Bateman DA, Wung JT, et al. Congenital diaphragmatic hernia in 120 infants treated consecutively with permissive hypercapnea/spontaneous respiration/elective repair. J Pediatr Surg 2002;37:357–66.
2. Wilson JM, Lund DP, Lillehei CW, et al. Congenital diaphragmatic hernia—a tale of two cities: the Boston experience. J Pediatr Surg 1997;32:401–5.
3. Mishalany HG, Nakada K, Woolley MM. Congenital diaphragmatic hernias: eleven years' experience. Arch Surg 1979;114:1118–23.
4. Stege G, Fenton A, Jaffray B. Nihilism in the 1990s: the true mortality of congenital diaphragmatic hernia. Pediatrics 2003;112:532–5.
5. Lally KP, Lally PA, Van Meurs KP, et al. Treatment evolution in high-risk congenital diaphragmatic hernia: ten years' experience with diaphragmatic agenesis. Ann Surg 2006;244:505–13.
6. Hirschl RB, Philip WF, Glick L, et al. A prospective, randomized pilot trial of perfluorocarbon-induced lung growth in newborns with congenital diaphragmatic hernia. J Pediatr Surg 2003;38:283–9 [discussion: 9].
7. Peralta CF, Sbragia L, Bennini JR, et al. Fetoscopic endotracheal occlusion for severe isolated diaphragmatic hernia: initial experience from a single clinic in Brazil. Fetal Diagn Ther 2011;29:71–7.
8. Ruano R, Duarte SA, Pimenta EJ, et al. Comparison between fetal endoscopic tracheal occlusion using a 1.0-mm fetoscope and prenatal expectant management in severe congenital diaphragmatic hernia. Fetal Diagn Ther 2011;29: 64–70.
9. Clark RH, Hardin WD Jr, Hirschl RB, et al. Current surgical management of congenital diaphragmatic hernia: a report from the Congenital Diaphragmatic Hernia Study Group. J Pediatr Surg 1998;33:1004–9.
10. Smith MJ, Paran TS, Quinn F, et al. The SIS extracellular matrix scaffold-preliminary results of use in congenital diaphragmatic hernia (CDH) repair. Pediatr Surg Int 2004;20:859–62.

11. Tsao K, Lally PA, Lally KP. Minimally invasive repair of congenital diaphragmatic hernia. J Pediatr Surg 2011;46:1158–64.
12. Arca MJ, Barnhart DC, Lelli JL Jr, et al. Early experience with minimally invasive repair of congenital diaphragmatic hernias: results and lessons learned. J Pediatr Surg 2003;38:1563–8.
13. Gander JW, Fisher JC, Gross ER, et al. Early recurrence of congenital diaphragmatic hernia is higher after thoracoscopic than open repair: a single institutional study. J Pediatr Surg 2011;46:1303–8.
14. Holcomb GW 3rd, Ostlie DJ, Miller KA. Laparoscopic patch repair of diaphragmatic hernias with Surgisis. J Pediatr Surg 2005;40:E1–5.
15. Keijzer R, van de Ven C, Vlot J, et al. Thoracoscopic repair in congenital diaphragmatic hernia: patching is safe and reduces the recurrence rate. J Pediatr Surg 2010;45:953–7.
16. Lansdale N, Alam S, Losty PD, et al. Neonatal endosurgical congenital diaphragmatic hernia repair: a systematic review and meta-analysis. Ann Surg 2010;252: 20–6.
17. Taskin M, Zengin K, Unal E, et al. Laparoscopic repair of congenital diaphragmatic hernias. Surg Endosc 2002;16:869.
18. McHoney M, Giacomello L, Nah SA, et al. Thoracoscopic repair of congenital diaphragmatic hernia: intraoperative ventilation and recurrence. J Pediatr Surg 2010;45:355–9.
19. Pacilli M, Pierro A, Kingsley C, et al. Absorption of carbon dioxide during laparoscopy in children measured using a novel mass spectrometric technique. Br J Anaesth 2006;97:215–9.
20. Bliss D, Matar M, Krishnaswami S. Should intraoperative hypercapnea or hypercarbia raise concern in neonates undergoing thoracoscopic repair of diaphragmatic hernia of Bochdalek? J Laparoendosc Adv Surg Tech A 2009; 19(Suppl 1):S55–8.
21. McHoney M, Corizia L, Eaton S, et al. Carbon dioxide elimination during laparoscopy in children is age dependent. J Pediatr Surg 2003;38:105–10 [discussion: 10].
22. McHoney MC, Corizia L, Eaton S, et al. Laparoscopic surgery in children is associated with an intraoperative hypermetabolic response. Surg Endosc 2006;20: 452–7.
23. Yang EY, Allmendinger N, Johnson SM, et al. Neonatal thoracoscopic repair of congenital diaphragmatic hernia: selection criteria for successful outcome. J Pediatr Surg 2005;40:1369–75.
24. Gourlay DM, Cassidy LD, Sato TT, et al. Beyond feasibility: a comparison of newborns undergoing thoracoscopic and open repair of congenital diaphragmatic hernias. J Pediatr Surg 2009;44:1702–7.
25. Kim AC, Bryner BS, Akay B, et al. Thoracoscopic repair of congenital diaphragmatic hernia in neonates: lessons learned. J Laparoendosc Adv Surg Tech A 2009;19:575–80.
26. Cho SD, Krishnaswami S, McKee JC, et al. Analysis of 29 consecutive thoracoscopic repairs of congenital diaphragmatic hernia in neonates compared to historical controls. J Pediatr Surg 2009;44:80–6 [discussion: 86].
27. Shah SR, Wishnew J, Barsness K, et al. Minimally invasive congenital diaphragmatic hernia repair: a 7-year review of one institution's experience. Surg Endosc 2009;23:1265–71.
28. Knight CG, Gidell KM, Lanning D, et al. Laparoscopic Morgagni hernia repair in children using robotic instruments. J Laparoendosc Adv Surg Tech A 2005;15: 482–6.

29. Meehan JJ, Sandler A. Robotic repair of a Bochdalek congenital diaphragmatic hernia in a small neonate: robotic advantages and limitations. J Pediatr Surg 2007;42:1757–60.

30. Slater BJ, Meehan JJ. Robotic repair of congenital diaphragmatic anomalies. J Laparoendosc Adv Surg Tech A 2009;19(Suppl 1):S123–7.

31. Tsao K, Allison ND, Harting MT, et al. Congenital diaphragmatic hernia in the preterm infant. Surgery 2010;148(2):404–10.

32. Grethel EJ, Cortes RA, Wagner AJ, et al. Prosthetic patches for congenital diaphragmatic hernia repair: Surgisis vs Gore-Tex. J Pediatr Surg 2006;41:29–33 [discussion: 29–33].

33. Hajer GF, van de Staak FH, de Haan AF, et al. Recurrent congenital diaphragmatic hernia; which factors are involved? Eur J Pediatr Surg 1998;8:329–33.

34. Moss RL, Chen CM, Harrison MR. Prosthetic patch durability in congenital diaphragmatic hernia: a long-term follow-up study. J Pediatr Surg 2001;36:152–4.

35. Loff S, Wirth H, Jester I, et al. Implantation of a cone-shaped double-fixed patch increases abdominal space and prevents recurrence of large defects in congenital diaphragmatic hernia. J Pediatr Surg 2005;40:1701–5.

36. Saltzman DA, Ennis JS, Mehall JR, et al. Recurrent congenital diaphragmatic hernia: a novel repair. J Pediatr Surg 2001;36:1768–9.

37. Riehle KJ, Magnuson DK, Waldhausen JH. Low recurrence rate after Gore-Tex/Marlex composite patch repair for posterolateral congenital diaphragmatic hernia. J Pediatr Surg 2007;42(11):1841–4.

38. Lally KP, Cheu HW, Vazquez WD. Prosthetic diaphragm reconstruction in the growing animal. J Pediatr Surg 1993;28:45–7.

39. St Peter SD, Valusek PA, Tsao K, et al. Abdominal complications related to type of repair for congenital diaphragmatic hernia. J Surg Res 2007;140:234–6.

40. Sandusky GE Jr, Badylak SF, Morff RJ, et al. Histologic findings after in vivo placement of small intestine submucosal vascular grafts and saphenous vein grafts in the carotid artery in dogs. Am J Pathol 1992;140:317–24.

41. Oelschlager BK, Barreca M, Chang L, et al. The use of small intestine submucosa in the repair of paraesophageal hernias: initial observations of a new technique. Am J Surg 2003;186:4–8.

42. Franklin ME Jr, Gonzalez JJ Jr, Michaelson RP, et al. Preliminary experience with new bioactive prosthetic material for repair of hernias in infected fields. Hernia 2002;6:171–4.

43. Mitchell IC, Garcia NM, Barber R, et al. Permacol: a potential biologic patch alternative in congenital diaphragmatic hernia repair. J Pediatr Surg 2008;43:2161–4.

44. Menon NG, Rodriguez ED, Byrnes CK, et al. Revascularization of human acellular dermis in full-thickness abdominal wall reconstruction in the rabbit model. Ann Plast Surg 2003;50:523–7.

45. Urita Y, Komuro H, Chen G, et al. Evaluation of diaphragmatic hernia repair using PLGA mesh-collagen sponge hybrid scaffold: an experimental study in a rat model. Pediatr Surg Int 2008;24:1041–5.

46. Sandoval JA, Lou D, Engum SA, et al. The whole truth: comparative analysis of diaphragmatic hernia repair using 4-ply vs 8-ply small intestinal submucosa in a growing animal model. J Pediatr Surg 2006;41:518–23.

47. Laituri CA, Garey CL, Valusek PA, et al. Outcome of congenital diaphragmatic hernia repair depending on patch type. Eur J Pediatr Surg 2010;20:363–5.

48. Kimber CP, Dunkley MP, Haddock G, et al. Patch incorporation in diaphragmatic hernia. J Pediatr Surg 2000;35:120–3.

49. Meeker IA Jr, Snyder WH Jr. Surgical management of diaphragmatic defects in the newborn infant. A report of twenty infants each less than one week old (1956-1961). Am J Surg 1962;104:196–203.
50. Simpson JS, Gossage JD. Use of abdominal wall muscle flap in repair of large congenital diaphragmatic hernia. J Pediatr Surg 1971;6:42–4.
51. Scaife ER, Johnson DG, Meyers RL, et al. The split abdominal wall muscle flap–a simple, mesh-free approach to repair large diaphragmatic hernia. J Pediatr Surg 2003;38:1748–51.
52. Brant-Zawadzki PB, Fenton SJ, Nichol PF, et al. The split abdominal wall muscle flap repair for large congenital diaphragmatic hernias on extracorporeal membrane oxygenation. J Pediatr Surg 2007;42:1047–50 [discussion: 1051].
53. Bianchi A, Doig CM, Cohen SJ. The reverse latissimus dorsi flap for congenital diaphragmatic hernia repair. J Pediatr Surg 1983;18:560–3.
54. Samarakkody U, Klaassen M, Nye B. Reconstruction of congenital agenesis of hemidiaphragm by combined reverse latissimus dorsi and serratus anterior muscle flaps. J Pediatr Surg 2001;36:1637–40.
55. Sydorak RM, Hoffman W, Lee H, et al. Reversed latissimus dorsi muscle flap for repair of recurrent congenital diaphragmatic hernia. J Pediatr Surg 2003;38:296–300 [discussion: 296–300].
56. Whetzel TP, Stokes RB, Greenholz SK, et al. Reconstruction of the toddler diaphragm in severe anterolateral congenital diaphragmatic hernia with the reverse latissimus dorsi flap. Ann Plast Surg 1997;39:615–9.
57. Barbosa RF, Rodrigues J, Correia-Pinto J, et al. Repair of a large congenital diaphragmatic defect with a reverse latissimus dorsi muscle flap. Microsurgery 2008;28:85–8.
58. Bekdash B, Singh B, Lakhoo K. Recurrent late complications following congenital diaphragmatic hernia repair with prosthetic patches: a case series. J Med Case Reports 2009;3:7237.
59. Ferrari G, Cusella-De Angelis G, Coletta M, et al. Muscle regeneration by bone marrow-derived myogenic progenitors. Science 1998;279:1528–30.
60. Rossi CA, Pozzobon M, Ditadi A, et al. Clonal characterization of rat muscle satellite cells: proliferation, metabolism and differentiation define an intrinsic heterogeneity. PLoS One 2010;5:e8523.
61. De Coppi P, Bartsch G Jr, Siddiqui MM, et al. Isolation of amniotic stem cell lines with potential for therapy. Nat Biotechnol 2007;25:100–6.
62. Fuchs JR, Kaviani A, Oh JT, et al. Diaphragmatic reconstruction with autologous tendon engineered from mesenchymal amniocytes. J Pediatr Surg 2004;39:834–8 [discussion: 838].
63. Turner CG, Klein JD, Steigman SA, et al. Preclinical regulatory validation of an engineered diaphragmatic tendon made with amniotic mesenchymal stem cells. J Pediatr Surg 2011;46:57–61.
64. Tsao K, Lally KP. The Congenital Diaphragmatic Hernia Study Group: a voluntary international registry. Semin Pediatr Surg 2008;17:90–7. CDH website. Available at: http://utsurg.uth.tmc.edu/pedisurgery/cdhsg/index.html. Accessed April 13, 2012.
65. Rygl M, Pycha K, Stranak Z, et al. Congenital diaphragmatic hernia: onset of respiratory distress and size of the defect: analysis of the outcome in 104 neonates. Pediatr Surg Int 2007;23:27–31.
66. Lally KP, Lally PA, Lasky RE, et al. Defect size determines survival in infants with congenital diaphragmatic hernia. Pediatrics 2007;120:e651–7.

67. Beck C, Alkasi O, Nikischin W, et al. Congenital diaphragmatic hernia, etiology and management, a 10-year analysis of a single center. Arch Gynecol Obstet 2008;277:55–63.
68. Fisher JC, Jefferson RA, Arkovitz MS, et al. Redefining outcomes in right congenital diaphragmatic hernia. J Pediatr Surg 2008;43:373–9.
69. Mallik K, Rodgers BM, McGahren ED. Congenital diaphragmatic hernia: experience in a single institution from 1978 through 1994. Ann Thorac Surg 1995;60:1331–5 [discussion: 1335–6].
70. Abdullah F, Zhang Y, Sciortino C, et al. Congenital diaphragmatic hernia: outcome review of 2,173 surgical repairs in US infants. Pediatr Surg Int 2009;25:1059–64.
71. Grushka JR, Laberge JM, Puligandla P, et al. Effect of hospital case volume on outcome in congenital diaphragmatic hernia: the experience of the Canadian Pediatric Surgery Network. J Pediatr Surg 2009;44:873–6.
72. Javid PJ, Jaksic T, Skarsgard ED, et al. Survival rate in congenital diaphragmatic hernia: the experience of the Canadian Neonatal Network. J Pediatr Surg 2004;39:657–60.
73. Lally KP, Paranka MS, Roden J, et al. Congenital diaphragmatic hernia. Stabilization and repair on ECMO. Ann Surg 1992;216:569–73.
74. Kinsella JP, Truog WE, Walsh WF, et al. Randomized, multicenter trial of inhaled nitric oxide and high-frequency oscillatory ventilation in severe, persistent pulmonary hypertension of the newborn. J Pediatr 1997;131:55–62.
75. Lotze A, Knight GR, Anderson KD, et al. Surfactant (beractant) therapy for infants with congenital diaphragmatic hernia on ECMO: evidence of persistent surfactant deficiency. J Pediatr Surg 1994;29:407–12.
76. Nio M, Haase G, Kennaugh J, et al. A prospective randomized trial of delayed versus immediate repair of congenital diaphragmatic hernia. J Pediatr Surg 1994;29:618–21.

Advances in Surgery for Abdominal Wall Defects
Gastroschisis and Omphalocele

Saleem Islam, MD, MPH

KEYWORDS

- Gastroschisis • Omphalocele • Prenatal diagnosis • Surgery • Neonatal

KEY POINTS

- Abdominal wall defects are comprised of 2 distinct entities, omphalocele and gastroschisis, which have very different management techniques and outcomes.
- Gastroschisis outcomes have improved dramatically over the past 4 decades, but still comprise the largest group of patients needing bowel transplant.
- Omphalocele outcomes remain poor overall despite many advances in care.
- Large omphaloceles are one of the most difficult things to manage in pediatric surgery and there is no standardized closure technique.
- There is a need to conduct multicenter prospective trials to better define groups of neonates with poor prognosis and to develop improved techniques to manage them.

Abdominal wall defects (AWDs) are the most common congenital surgical problem in fetuses and neonates. The incidence of these defects has steadily increased over the past few decades due to rising numbers of gastroschisis. Most of these anomalies are diagnosed prenatally and then managed at a center with readily available pediatric surgical, neonatology, and high-risk obstetric support. While commonly lumped together, omphaloceles and gastroschisis are distinct anomalies that have different management and outcomes; therefore, they will be considered separately. There have been several recent advances in the care of patients with AWDs, both in the fetus and the newborn, which will be discussed in this article.

OMPHALOCELE
Termination and the Hidden Mortality

Omphaloceles have an incidence of 1 case per 1100 population in fetuses at around 14 to 18 weeks gestation, yet the number of live born is 1 case per 4000 to 6000 infants.[1,2] These defects have a very high rate of termination of pregnancy (30%–52%)

Pediatric Surgery, Department of Surgery, University of Florida College of Medicine, Post Office Box 100119, 1600 SW Archer Road, Gainesville, FL 32607, USA
E-mail address: saleem.islam@surgery.ufl.edu

Clin Perinatol 39 (2012) 375–386
doi:10.1016/j.clp.2012.04.008
0095-5108/12/$ – see front matter © 2012 Elsevier Inc. All rights reserved.

due to the presence of associated anomalies in addition to attrition (fetal demise, spontaneous abortion –(5%–10%) above and beyond termination.[3,4] Some reviews state that the termination request rate for omphaloceles may be as high as 83%.[4] Most reports differentiate isolated omphalocele from those with other associated defects, due to the fact that survival is considered to be highly dependent on the presence and severity of these anomalies (isolated omphalocele has a survival rate of as high as 96%).[5,6] Data suggest that prenatal ultrasound and karyotyping are able to identify 60% to 70% of the associated defects that become apparent postnatally.[6] In 2 recent series, survival for neonates with isolated omphaloceles and those with nonisolated omphaloceles that were not picked up during prenatal evaluation were found to be similar.[7,8] However, these same studies showed that the overall survival of fetuses with omphalocele was between 23% and 52%. Thus, when one analyzes the survival in live born neonates, one is already dealing with a selected group of patients, with improved likelihood of survival.

Prenatal Diagnosis, Counseling, and Therapy

Prenatal diagnosis in omphaloceles is usually made in the late first trimester to midsecond trimester by ultrasound screening or as part of a positive triple test with elevated maternal α fetoprotein.[8] As opposed to gastroschisis, these fetuses undergo further tests to look for associated anomalies or chromosomal abnormalities. Other anomalies are found in up to 80% of fetuses with normal karyotype, while chromosomal defects are noted in approximately 49% (mostly trisomy 13, 18, or 21).[8] A recent study that collated all recent publications detailing the associated defects in AWD patients noted anomalies that involved every organ system, while a study from the Netherlands indicated that only 14% of omphaloceles were truly isolated.[6,9] Prenatal screening in omphalocele fetuses needs to have a detailed evaluation of the cardiac system (14%–47%) and central nervous system (3%–33%), as severe defects may lead to a serious discussion on termination of pregnancy.[9] However, fully one-third of fetuses considered to be isolated have multiple associated defects detected postnatally.[6] This is important information for discussions that high-risk pregnancy teams have with prospective parents with an omphalocele fetus (which are centered on the key question of postnatal outcome and morbidity). Recently, there has been some attention directed toward developing a reliable sonographic predictor of postnatal morbidity and survival.[10–12] Previous estimates have relied on defining a giant omphalocele; however, this has not been a reliable predictor for a number of reasons. First, the definition of a giant omphalocele in a fetus is variable, with some studies using a 4 cm diameter or 5 cm diameter criterion, and others defining it based on the presence or absence of liver outside the abdomen.[13] Second, these studies have shown no significant impact on the diagnosis of either extracorporeal liver or a giant omphalocele in postnatal survival and therefore have not been useful in guiding families.[13] In the past few years, some investigators have studied ratios between the greatest omphalocele diameter compared with abdominal circumference (O/AC), femur length (O/FL), and head circumference (O/HC), and attempted to correlate that with postnatal morbidity and mortality.[13,14] Of these, potentially the most useful may be the O/HC, which if 0.21 or greater had 84% sensitivity and 58% specificity at predicting the need for staged versus primary closure and respiratory insufficiency.[13] These data were obtained in retrospective studies and need to be verified prospectively before becoming standards for predicting postnatal outcome. There are currently no routine fetal interventions that are performed either experimentally or in people for omphaloceles specifically other than amniocentesis for karyotype.

The timing of delivery of an omphalocele is not controversial, and most infants are born at term unless there are complicating features such as polyhydraminos. Preterm delivery is not recommended. The route of delivery, however, is not a settled issue, with proponents of vaginal birth as well as cesarean section. In large defects in which most of the liver is extra-abdominal, concern for hepatic injury during vaginal delivery prompts a cesarean section.[5] To date there has been no study that advocates 1 method over the other, and there are numerous reports of safe delivery of omphalocele patients vaginally.[15]

Management of the Large or Giant Defect

In general, the surgical management of omphaloceles for the small- or even medium-sized (2–4 cm) defects is fairly standard and involves primary closure with good surgical outcomes. In these cases, the survival and morbidity are dependent upon the associated defects. Interestingly, small defects, especially those in the central location (as opposed to hypogastric or epigastric locations), have a higher incidence of associated anomalies and chromosomal issues.[8] Most of the larger defects that survive to birth do not have lethal associated defects, and present some of the most challenging problems for pediatric surgeons and neonatologists.

In a recent survey performed by a Dutch group of surgeons, authors of reports discussing closure of giant omphaloceles (1967–2009) were asked to see if they are still performing the same repair, or whether they have modified their techniques. They concluded that over a 30 - year period there has been no completely accepted technique to treat giant omphaloceles and that, in general, 2 methods have persisted, staged or delayed closure of the defect.[16] This study did not address the issue with the previous mentioned heterogeneity of the definition of a giant omphalocele, similar to the prenatal ultrasonographic definition issues. Some authors use size alone; others consider the presence or absence of liver, while others use an estimate of the amount of intestinal contents (all or partial). Still others have used a combination of liver and intestines.[17,18] This has resulted in an inability to truly combine the literature and arrive at a consensus.

Most data on the surgical aspects of omphalocele closure are from small single institution studies or case reports detailing a specific technique that was used. As mentioned previously, they may be broadly classified into non operative (delayed repair), or staged methods.[18] In addition to these methods, there are several reports of primary closure of a giant omphalocele shortly after birth with good results.[17,19] In a report from London, 12 of 24 cases of large defects had an immediate repair performed without any mortality, and compared with the remaining cases, had a shorter ventilator requirement and time to attain full feeds.[19] However, this trial was not prospective, and there was significant selection bias toward the full -term and normal birth weight neonates for immediate repair. In addition, the definition of large was not uniformly applied. Most cases of large defects are not considered amenable to immediate repair due to the lack of abdominal domain.[18]

Nonoperative techniques have in common the use of an agent that allows an eschar to form over the intact amnion sac, which epithelializes over time, leaving a ventral hernia that will likely require repair later in life.[18] This method has been employed when the surgeon considers the defect too large to allow for safe primary repair, or if the neonate has significant concurrent cardiac or respiratory issues that would preclude an attempt at surgery. This is not a new concept, having evolved from the time of Gross, who described using skin flaps in 1948, and others who used alcohol as a topical agent in 1899.[20] Concerns in large isolated defects are that an initial repair without having abdominal domain for the organs would result in potential life-threatening abdominal compartment syndrome or inability to provide skin coverage and. Therefore, this approach would not be ideal. Initial reports described mercurochrome, alcohol, and silver nitrate as the eschar-producing agents, which were very effective, but associated with toxicity and abandoned.[20] Subsequently, there have been reports of a number of agents used, including silver sulfadiazine, povidone–iodine solution, silver impregnated dressings, neomycin, and polymixin/bacitracin ointments.[20–24] The eschar and epithelialization may take over 4 to 10 weeks to complete, and in some cases, patients complete the process after discharge. There are also reports that combine the use of an agent listed previously with compression dressing, which helps in reducing the contents in the abdomen and facilitates closure.[25] In some cases, there is no need for surgical closure, as the defect contracts and closes similar to an umbilical hernia; however, most patients will eventually require closure of a ventral hernia defect, which is usually performed between 1 and 5 years of age. The repair is performed via either primary fascial closure, autologous repair with component separation, or use of a mesh repair.[21,26,27] Each has been reported with success; however, the number of patients in each report is small, and, without prospective studies, the failures are usually not reported. In some cases, innovative techniques have been used to recreate the abdominal domain including the use of tissue expanders in the abdomen that are gradually increased in size.[28] While the initial reports of the staged Gross operation had significant mortality and morbidity, current results are much better, with very few deaths reported.[21]

Staged closure in the neonatal period involves the use of a variety of different techniques to obtain closure with multiple procedures. These can be classified into methods that use the existing amnion sac with serial inversion and those in which the sac is excised and replaced with mesh and then closed over time. Amnion inversion allows gradual reduction of the sac and, when completely involuted, the sac is excised and either a primary closure is performed or mesh is used.[29] There are several reports that detail different methods of mesh closure, each with the similar goal of obtaining skin and fascial apposition. This may be achieved by excision of the mesh sequentially, allowing for native fascial closure. Alternatively, mesh may be left in situ with skin coverage on top.[30] Some authors have advocated the use of biologic mesh that becomes incorporated and may have less recurrent hernia formation.[31,32] Vacuum-assisted closure of these defects has also been described, as has a novel external skin closure system.[33,34] Again, it is difficult to truly compare the series, as the definition of size of the defect is not uniform.

A large, prenatally ruptured omphalocele is a special situation that represents one of the most difficult problems in pediatric surgery. The goal in repair of these unique situations is to obtain coverage of the exposed abdominal viscera, which is challenging and, aside from a few case reports, there is not much experience. There is 1 small series that has good outcome in terms of survival, but there is a high incidence of intestinal fistulas, sepsis, and pulmonary hypoplasia that can lead to poor outcomes.[35]

Outcomes in Omphaloceles

As has been discussed, the outcomes in this defect may be looked at in 2 ways: survival of fetuses diagnosed with omphalocele, or in those who are live born.[17] Multiple studies have documented survival of less than 20% to 50% in prenatally diagnosed cases (including termination).[8] A report from London indicated that 90% of cases with prenatal diagnosis reached the point of undergoing surgical repair.[36] Studies looking at survival postnatally document a close association with the presence of defects and chromosomal anomalies.[5,36,37] Going beyond survival alone, there are several issues that lead to continuing morbidity. Pulmonary hypoplasia can be severe in these neonates and may require prolonged mechanical ventilation and tracheostomy.[38] However, long-term follow-up in a cohort of older children documented normal lung volumes and oxygen consumption.[39] Gastroesophageal reflux is also common, as well as failure to thrive, and these are significant issues that require long-term therapy and a high incidence of fundoplication and nutritional support.[37,40] One long-term concern in patients with giant omphaloceles is the cosmetic appearance of their abdomen and the missing umbilicus.[41] Outside of these few studies, there are few data on the long-term outcomes in infants with omphalocele, and the use of multicenter registries would be beneficial in understanding the true impact of these defects and the cost associated with them.

GASTROSCHISIS
Prenatal Therapy

Most gastroschisis patients are diagnosed and identified prenatally and are delivered at a center with the ability to care for the neonate. Most are diagnosed in the early to mid-second trimester, providing ample time for consideration of any prenatal interventions designed to improve postnatal outcomes. The issues that lead to intestinal damage and prolonged dysmotility are thought to be the result of interactions between the bowel serosa and the amniotic fluid, and in particular the meconium and other waste products in the fluid.[42–44] To ameliorate the effects of this interaction, studies in small and large animal models have suggested a benefit to altering the amniotic fluid environment.[44–46] Three interventions have been attempted: (1) amniotic fluid removal and exchange with physiologic fluid, (2) amniotic fluid supplementation in cases of oligohydramnios, and (3) amniotic instillation of furosemide to induce fetal diuresis.[43,47–49] Each of the interventions showed promise in animal models, with reduction in the intestinal damage as measured by the thickness of the peel, number of interstitial cells of Cajal, and inflammatory markers. However, it is unclear whether these interventions can result in any long-term benefit. There have been a few instances of human amniotic fluid exchange as well as amnio infusion for oligohydramnios in the setting of gastroschisis, but the number of patients is too few to make any conclusions.[50,51] In 1 small study of 10 gastroschisis patients compared with controls, there was a reduced hospital length of stay when compared with controls, but no other variables were reported.[52] Thus, prenatal therapy holds promise, but with a current survival rate of over 90% in cases without any intervention, safety issues may limit its usefulness and adoption.

Ultrasonographic Markers of Concern

Since a report in 2001 that recommended stratification of gastroschisis cases into complicated and simple, there has been growing realization that these 2 classifications may actually be different disease conditions with different outcomes.[53] The authors defined complicated gastroschisis as one in which there is a bowel atresia; perforation; ischemia or necrosis; or bowel loss that has occurred in utero. Efforts have been directed at accurately predicting which fetuses will develop complicated problems. Initial reports considered the appearance of the intestine and the stomach, but recently focus has been directed to the diameter of the loops of intestine that are contained within the abdomen. Alfaraj and colleagues[54] made note that gastric dilation predicted the presence of meconium-stained fluid, but no other adverse outcome. Lato and the group from Dusseldorf found improved predictive capability of ultrasound when both intestinal dilation and gestational age were noted, and they were able to correlate bowel atresia with dilation of greater than 10 mm noted before 30 weeks gestation.[55] Contro and colleagues and Huh and colleagues identified intestinal damage in 29% and 37% of fetuses respectively using greater than 6 mm diameter as a cutoff.[56,57] The studies are still plagued by inconsistent use of the measurement

(>6–>20 mm) and the time in gestation that it is noted; therefore, the usefulness is controversial.[58] Further work with larger multicenter prospective studies is needed to refine the ability to predict intestinal damage and complex gastroschisis and improve prenatal counseling.[58]

Route and Timing of Delivery

The issues of when and how to deliver a fetus with an AWD, especially gastroschisis, remain controversial despite many advances in the past few decades in the understanding of AWD.[15] Most gastroschisis fetuses are born prematurely around 34 to 36 weeks gestation and are small for gestational age due to significant intrauterine growth retardation (IUGR).[59] There was significant interest in having these babies delivered prematurely via induction or cesarean at 34 to 36 weeks to limit the duration of time that the intestines were exposed to amniotic fluid, based on data from animal studies. Additionally, by performing a scheduled delivery, the neonate could be delivered at a facility where appropriate resources were present to care for the newborn. One prospective, randomized trial in the United Kingdom was designed to study outcomes from elective preterm delivery at 36 weeks versus undergoing spontaneous labor, using an intent-to-treat strategy, and found no benefit to preterm delivery.[60] Opposing evidence came from a prospective, but nonrandomized study at the Mayo clinic involving only 16 patients with elective delivery at 34 weeks, which reported reduced total parenteral nutrition (TPN) duration, decreased length of hospital stay, and a higher rate of primary closure of the gastroschisis compared with a historical cohort.[61] Another retrospective review from Mannheim noted that elective cesarean section before 36 weeks led to earlier closure of the defect and enteral feeding,[62] while Vegunta and colleagues[63] reported benefits from planned cesarean section at 36 to 38 weeks with higher rates of primary repair. Two further reports from Pittsburgh looking at 75 cases of gastroschisis, and Portugal with 65 patients, found that patients electively delivered early had no difference in the appearance of the bowel compared with normal deliveries, but had a longer hospital length of stay. As a result, these authors advocated against preterm delivery.[64,65] The data are mixed, but the evidence falls to the side of allowing spontaneous delivery close to term as opposed to elective preterm birth in the setting of gastroschisis.

Abdel-Latif, and colleagues,[66] reporting on behalf of the Australia New Zealand Neonatal Network, compared the short term outcomes in babies with gastroschisis born via vaginal versus elective/emergency cesarean section. Fifty-four percent were delivered vaginally, and there was no difference in any parameter of short-term outcome between the groups. The group from Montreal published retrospective series and, again, found no benefit to cesarean delivery in gastroschisis.[67] In 2000, How and colleagues[68] reported their experience with 102 infants with an AWD and recommended cesarean section for obstetric indications only. In another retrospective review, authors from Kansas City noted a significant trend over time (30-year period) toward cesarean section,[69] despite a lack of evidence to suggest its benefit. Segel published a systematic review regarding mode of delivery and AWD, and, again, found no advantage to a cesarean section.[15] The evidence would suggest that in the absence of obstetric indications, most gastroschisis fetuses should be allowed to deliver vaginally.

Silo or Immediate Closure?

Another point of contention in the care of gastroschisis patients is the method used to close the defect. Schuster first described the creation of a silo for patients in whom there was lack of domain for the viscera (viscero abdominal disproportion). The silo was sewn to the fascia and allowed a gradual return of the viscera to the abdomen.

In the past couple of decades, the preformed, spring-loaded silo has made this method easier and has become popular as a form of initial closure.[70] The debate is whether patients have improved outcomes with either immediate reduction and closure or a delayed closure after a silo and gradual reduction. Retrospective reports have argued the benefits of each method, citing benefits with regard to ventilator time, time to full feeds, length of stay, and complication rates such as abdominal compartment syndrome, bowel ischemia, and necrotizing eterocolitis (NEC).[71–74] Pastor and colleagues[75] performed a multicenter, randomized, prospective trial comparing outcomes between silo and immediate closure. While they could not meet their accrual goals, they showed no significant difference between either group for most outcomes, other than duration of ventilation, which tended to be less in the silo group. A Canadian Association of Pediatric Surgeons network (CAPSnet) study published in 2008 reviewed the experience in the first 99 cases of gastroschisis in Canada and noted that there was no difference in overall outcome in silo versus immediate closure other than an increased length of stay and duration of TPN usage in the silo group that likely reflected the observational nature of the study.[76] In 2011, a cooperative, observational trial from the United Kingdom that captured 77% (301 of 393) of all gastroschisis births over a 17-month period noted that patients who had a silo placed took 5 days longer to reach full enteral feeds and had a higher risk of intestinal failure when compared with immediate closure.[77] However, this was a nonselected group of patients, and the authors cautioned in overinterpreting these data, as patients who had a silo were likely to have had more viscera outside the abdomen. They did suggest performing a prospective study to address this question. Final closure technique has also been debated recently, with groups reporting successful nonoperative and sutureless final closure for either the immediate reduction or silo patients.[78,79] Techniques for this have involved the use of the umbilical cord tissue and dressing changes and Steri Strips with vacuum-assisted closure.[80,81] Advantages of this method are the avoidance of anesthesia for bedside closure as well as improved cosmetic results.

Management of Complicated Gastroschisis

Molik and colleagues[53] published an article in 2001 in which they strongly advocated for risk adjustment in gastroschisis to allow better comparison of patients and outcomes. This was borne out by 2 administrative database reviews from the United States that supported and validated the classification of gastroschisis into complex and simple based on the presence of bowel atresia, perforation, ischemia, or prenatal loss of intestine with short bowel syndrome.[82,83] Outcomes are quite different between these 2 groups, and long-term morbidity is almost entirely confined to the complex group and associated short bowel syndrome, liver failure due to prolonged parenteral nutrition, and sepsis. Most reviews estimate 5% to 15% of gastroschisis cases are complex, and these patients predictably have a longer length of stay, increased TPN usage, and increased costs as compared with the simple cases.[84] The most common type of complex gastroschisis is a concomitant bowel atresia, seen in up to 15% of patients. Bowel atresia management depends upon the condition of the bowel and the infant.[85] In most cases, the thickness and extent of the peel will not allow immediate anastomosis. Therefore, the options are to reduce the viscera and perform repair in 3 to 5 weeks, allowing the intestines to normalize, or in more distal atresias, to create an ostomy that would allow for enteral feedings before definitive repair.[86] The prolonged time on parenteral nutrition is responsible for the morbidity due to sepsis and cholestatic liver disease. Modern management of patients with short bowel at specialized centers may help improve survival for this group of patients. Efforts at prenatal detection of this group of patients, as discussed previously, would help in counseling parents.

Outcomes

Outcomes in gastroschisis have changed dramatically in the past 4 decades, with the advent of improved neonatal intensive care unit, surgical, obstetric, and nutritional care. Overall, survival went from 50% to 60% in the 1960s to greater than 90% currently. Long-term issues are rare in patients without bowel injury, and most infants catch up in growth with their non-AWD cohorts within a few years.[2] IUGR in gastroschisis does not have significant impact on outcome. Despite having malrotation, the incidence of volvulus is rare in gastroschisis, and a Ladd procedure is rarely required. Undescended testicles are noted in 15% to 30% of males with gastroschisis, with a large number having extra-abdominal gonads at birth. Fifty percent or more of these testicles will descend spontaneously by 12 months of age, while the remainder will require an orchiopexy at that point.[87] Simply replacing the testicle in the abdomen at the time of final closure is recommended. The improved survival and diminished morbidity from gastroschisis may be noted from the fact that up to 60% of children will report psychological stress at the absence of a normal umbilicus, and this may be the most prevalent long-term issue requiring reconstruction in some cases.[88]

SUMMARY

AWDs are comprised of 2 distinct entities, omphalocele and gastroschisis, that have very different management techniques and outcomes. Overall, survival has improved considerably, especially for gastroschisis. However, there is a need to conduct multicenter prospective trials to better define groups of neonates with poor prognosis and to develop improved techniques to manage them.

REFERENCES

1. Blazer S, Zimmer EZ, Gover A, et al. Fetal omphalocele detected early in pregnancy: associated anomalies and outcomes. Radiology 2004;232:191–5.
2. Christison-Lagay ER, Kelleher CM, Langer JC. Neonatal abdominal wall defects. Semin Fetal Neonatal Med 2011;16:164–72.
3. Fratelli N, Papageorghiou AT, Bhide A, et al. Outcome of antenatally diagnosed abdominal wall defects. Ultrasound Obstet Gynecol 2007;30:266–70.
4. Garne E, Loane M, Dolk H. Gastrointestinal malformations: impact of prenatal diagnosis on gestational age at birth. Paediatr Perinat Epidemiol 2007;21:370–5.
5. Heider AL, Strauss RA, Kuller JA. Omphalocele: clinical outcomes in cases with normal karyotypes. Am J Obstet Gynecol 2004;190:135–41.
6. Cohen-Overbeek TE, Tong WH, Hatzmann TR, et al. Omphalocele: comparison of outcome following prenatal or postnatal diagnosis. Ultrasound Obstet Gynecol 2010;36:687–92.
7. Kominiarek MA, Zork N, Pierce SM, et al. Perinatal outcome in the live-born infant with prenatally diagnosed omphalocele. Am J Perinatol 2011;28:627–34.
8. Brantberg A, Blaas HG, Haugen SE, et al. Characteristics and outcome of 90 cases of fetal omphalocele. Ultrasound Obstet Gynecol 2005;26:527–37.
9. Frolov P, Alali J, Klein MD. Clinical risk factors for gastroschisis and omphalocele in humans: a review of the literature. Pediatr Surg Int 2010;26:1135–48.
10. Nicholas SS, Stamilio DM, Dicke JM, et al. Predicting adverse neonatal outcomes in fetuses with abdominal wall defects using prenatal risk factors. Am J Obstet Gynecol 2009;201:383.e1–6.
11. Kamata S, Usui N, Sawai T, et al. Prenatal detection of pulmonary hypoplasia in giant omphalocele. Pediatr Surg Int 2008;24(1):107–11.

12. Hidaka N, Tsukimori K, Hojo S, et al. Correlation between the presence of liver herniation and perinatal outcome in prenatally diagnosed fetal omphalocele. J Perinat Med 2009;37:66–71.
13. Montero FJ, Simpson LL, Brady PC, et al. Fetal omphalocele ratios predict outcomes in prenatally diagnosed omphalocele. Am J Obstet Gynecol 2011;205:284.e1–7.
14. Kleinrouweler CE, Kuijper CF, van Zalen-Sprock MM, et al. Characteristics and outcome and the omphalocele circumference/abdominal circumference ratio in prenatally diagnosed fetal omphalocele. Fetal Diagn Ther 2011;30:60–9.
15. Segel SY, Marder SJ, Parry S, et al. Fetal abdominal wall defects and mode of delivery: a systematic review. Obstet Gynecol 2001;98:867–73.
16. van Eijck FC, Aronson DA, Hoogeveen YL, et al. Past and current surgical treatment of giant omphalocele: outcome of a questionnaire sent to authors. J Pediatr Surg 2011;46:482–8.
17. Islam S. Clinical care outcomes in abdominal wall defects. Curr Opin Pediatr 2008;20:305–10.
18. Mortellaro VE, St Peter SD, Fike FB, et al. Review of the evidence on the closure of abdominal wall defects. Pediatr Surg Int 2011;27(4):391–7.
19. Rijhwani A, Davenport M, Dawrant M, et al. Definitive surgical management of antenatally diagnosed exomphalos. J Pediatr Surg 2005;40:516–22.
20. Whitehouse JS, Gourlay DM, Masonbrink AR, et al. Conservative management of giant omphalocele with topical povidone-iodine and its effect on thyroid function. J Pediatr Surg 2010;45:1192–7.
21. Lee SL, Beyer TD, Kim SS, et al. Initial nonoperative management and delayed closure for treatment of giant omphaloceles. J Pediatr Surg 2006;41:1846–9.
22. Almond S, Reyna R, Barganski N, et al. Nonoperative management of a giant omphalocele using a silver impregnated hydrofiber dressing: a case report. J Pediatr Surg 2010;45:1546–9.
23. Wakhlu A, Wakhlu AK. The management of exomphalos. J Pediatr Surg 2000;35:73–6.
24. Lewis N, Kolimarala V, Lander A. Conservative management of exomphalos major with silver dressings: are they safe? J Pediatr Surg 2010;45:2438–9.
25. Hatch EI Jr, Baxter R. Surgical options in the management of large omphaloceles. Am J Surg 1987;153:449–52.
26. Pereira RM, Tatsuo ES, Simoes e Silva AC, et al. New method of surgical delayed closure of giant omphaloceles: Lazaro da Silva's technique. J Pediatr Surg 2004;39:1111–5.
27. van Eijck FC, de Blaauw I, Bleichrodt RP, et al. Closure of giant omphaloceles by the abdominal wall component separation technique in infants. J Pediatr Surg 2008;43:246–50.
28. De Ugarte DA, Asch MJ, Hedrick MH, et al. The use of tissue expanders in the closure of a giant omphalocele. J Pediatr Surg 2004;39:613–5.
29. de Lorimer AA, Adzick NS, Harrison MR. Amnion inversion in the treatment of giant omphalocele. J Pediatr Surg 1991;26:804–7.
30. Pacilli M, Spitz L, Kiely EM, et al. Staged repair of giant omphalocele in the neonatal period. J Pediatr Surg 2005;40:785–8.
31. Kapfer SA, Keshen TH. The use of human acellular dermis in the operative management of giant omphalocele. J Pediatr Surg 2006;41:216–20.
32. Alaish SM, Strauch ED. The use of Alloderm in the closure of a giant omphalocele. J Pediatr Surg 2006;41:e37–9.
33. Baird R, Gholoum S, Laberge JM, et al. Management of a giant omphalocele with an external skin closure system. J Pediatr Surg 2010;45:E17–20.

34. Kilbride KE, Cooney DR, Custer MD. Vacuum-assisted closure: a new method for treating patients with giant omphalocele. J Pediatr Surg 2006;41:212–5.

35. Bawazir OA, Wong A, Sigalet DL. Absorbable mesh and skin flaps or grafts in the management of ruptured giant omphalocele. J Pediatr Surg 2003;38:725–8.

36. Lakasing L, Cicero S, Davenport M, et al. Current outcome of antenatally diagnosed exomphalos: an 11 year review. J Pediatr Surg 2006;41:1403–6.

37. Biard JM, Wilson RD, Johnson MP, et al. Prenatally diagnosed giant omphaloceles: short- and long-term outcomes. Prenat Diagn 2004;24:434–9.

38. Edwards EA, Broome S, Green S, et al. Long-term respiratory support in children with giant omphalocele. Anaesth Intensive Care 2007;35:94–8.

39. Zaccara A, Iacobelli BD, Calzolari A, et al. Cardiopulmonary performances in young children and adolescents born with large abdominal wall defects. J Pediatr Surg 2003;38:478–81.

40. Koivusalo A, Rintala R, Lindahl H. Gastroesophageal reflux in children with a congenital abdominal wall defect. J Pediatr Surg 1999;34:1127–9.

41. van Eijck FC, Hoogeveen YL, van Weel C, et al. Minor and giant omphalocele: long-term outcomes and quality of life. J Pediatr Surg 2009;44:1355–9.

42. Api A, Olguner M, Hakguder G, et al. Intestinal damage in gastroschisis correlates with the concentration of intraamniotic meconium. J Pediatr Surg 2001;36:1811–5.

43. Hakguder G, Olguner M, Gurel D, et al. Induction of fetal diuresis with intra-amniotic furosemide injection reduces intestinal damage in a rat model of gastroschisis. Eur J Pediatr Surg 2011;21:183–7.

44. Olguner M, Akgur FM, Api A, et al. The effects of intra-amniotic human neonatal urine and meconium on the intestines of the chick embryo with gastroschisis. J Pediatr Surg 2000;35:458–61.

45. Olguner M, Hakguder G, Ates O, et al. Urinary trypsin inhibitor present in fetal urine prevents intraamniotic meconium-induced intestinal damage in gastroschisis. J Pediatr Surg 2006;41:1407–12.

46. Luton D, de Lagausie P, Guibourdenche J, et al. Influence of amnioinfusion in a model of in utero created gastroschisis in the pregnant ewe. Fetal Diagn Ther 2000;15:224–8.

47. Aktug T, Ucan B, Olguner M, et al. Amnio-allantoic fluid exchange for the prevention of intestinal damage in gastroschisis. III: determination of the waste products removed by exchange. Eur J Pediatr Surg 1998;8:326–8.

48. Aktug T, Demir N, Akgur FM, et al. Pretreatment of gastroschisis with transabdominal amniotic fluid exchange. Obstet Gynecol 1998;91:821–3.

49. Dommergues M, Ansker Y, Aubry MC, et al. Serial transabdominal amnio-infusion in the management of gastroschisis with severe oligohydramnios. J Pediatr Surg 1996;31:1297–9.

50. Luton D, Guibourdenche J, Vuillard E, et al. Prenatal management of gastroschisis: the place of the amnioexchange procedure. Clin Perinatol 2003;30:551–72.

51. Luton D, de Lagausie P, Guibourdenche J, et al. Effect of amnioinfusion on the outcome of prenatally diagnosed gastroschisis. Fetal Diagn Ther 1999;14:152–5.

52. Midrio P, Stefanutti G, Mussap M, et al. Amnioexchange for fetuses with gastroschisis: is it effective? J Pediatr Surg 2007;42:777–82.

53. Molik KA, Gingalewski CA, West KW, et al. Gastroschisis: a plea for risk categorization. J Pediatr Surg 2001;36:51–5.

54. Alfaraj MA, Ryan G, Langer JC, et al. Does gastric dilation predict adverse perinatal or surgical outcome in fetuses with gastroschisis? Ultrasound Obstet Gynecol 2011;37:202–6.

55. Lato K, Poellmann M, Knippel AJ, et al. Fetal gastroschisis: a comparison of second- vs. third-trimester bowel dilatation for predicting bowel atresia and neonatal outcomes. Ultraschall Med 2011. [Epub ahead of print].

56. Huh NG, Hirose S, Goldstein RB. Prenatal intra-abdominal bowel dilation is associated with postnatal gastrointestinal complications in fetuses with gastroschisis. Am J Obstet Gynecol 2010;202:396, e1–6.

57. Contro E, Fratelli N, Okoye B, et al. Prenatal ultrasound in the prediction of bowel obstruction in infants with gastroschisis. Ultrasound Obstet Gynecol 2010;35: 702–7.

58. Tower C, Ong SS, Ewer AK, et al. Prognosis in isolated gastroschisis with bowel dilatation: a systematic review. Arch Dis Child 2009;94:F268–74.

59. Lausman AY, Langer JC, Tai M, et al. Gastroschisis: what is the average gestational age of spontaneous delivery? J Pediatr Surg 2007;42:1816–21.

60. Logghe HL, Mason GC, Thornton JG, et al. A randomized controlled trial of elective preterm delivery of fetuses with gastroschisis. J Pediatr Surg 2005;40: 1726–31.

61. Moir CR, Ramsey PS, Ogburn PL, et al. A prospective trial of elective preterm delivery for fetal gastroschisis. Am J Perinatol 2004;21:289–94.

62. Hadidi A, Subotic U, Goeppl M, et al. Early elective cesarean delivery before 36 weeks vs late spontaneous delivery in infants with gastroschisis. J Pediatr Surg 2008;43:1342–6.

63. Vegunta RK, Wallace LJ, Leonardi MR, et al. Perinatal management of gastroschisis: analysis of a newly established clinical pathway. J Pediatr Surg 2005;40: 528–34.

64. Soares H, Silva A, Rocha G, et al. Gastroschisis: preterm or term delivery? Clinics (Sao Paulo, Brazil) 2010;65:139–42.

65. Ergün O, Barksdale E, Ergün FS, et al. The timing of delivery of infants with gastroschisis influences outcome. J Pediatr Surg 2005;40:424–8.

66. Abdel-Latif ME, Bolisetty S, Abeywardana S, et al. Mode of delivery and neonatal survival of infants with gastroschisis in Australia and New Zealand. J Pediatr Surg 2008;43:1685–90.

67. Puligandla PS, Janvier A, Flageole H, et al. Routine cesarean delivery does not improve the outcome of infants with gastroschisis. J Pediatr Surg 2004;39:742–5.

68. How HY, Harris BJ, Pietrantoni M, et al. Is vaginal delivery preferable to elective cesarean delivery in fetuses with a known ventral wall defect? Am J Obstet Gynecol 2000;182:1527–34.

69. Snyder CL, St Peter SD. Trends in mode of delivery for gastroschisis infants. Am J Perinatol 2005;22:391–6.

70. Kidd JN Jr, Jackson RJ, Smith SD, et al. Evolution of staged versus primary closure of gastroschisis. Ann Surg 2003;237:759–64.

71. Allotey J, Davenport M, Njere I, et al. Benefit of preformed silos in the management of gastroschisis. Pediatr Surg Int 2007;23:1065–9.

72. Owen A, Marven S, Jackson L, et al. Experience of bedside preformed silo staged reduction and closure for gastroschisis. J Pediatr Surg 2006;41:1830–5.

73. Banyard D, Ramones T, Phillips SE, et al. Method to our madness: an 18-year retrospective analysis on gastroschisis closure. J Pediatr Surg 2010;45:579–84.

74. Jensen AR, Waldhausen JH, Kim SS. The use of a spring-loaded silo for gastroschisis: impact on practice patterns and outcomes. Arch Surg 2009;144:516–9.

75. Pastor AC, Phillips JD, Fenton SJ, et al. Routine use of a SILASTIC spring-loaded silo for infants with gastroschisis: a multicenter randomized controlled trial. J Pediatr Surg 2008;43:1807–12.

76. Skarsgard ED, Claydon J, Bouchard S, et al. Canadian Pediatric Surgical Network: a population-based pediatric surgery network and database for analyzing surgical birth defects. The first 100 cases of gastroschisis. J Pediatr Surg 2008;43:30–4.

77. Bradnock TJ, Marven S, Owen A, et al. Gastroschisis: one-year outcomes from national cohort study. BMJ 2011;343:d6749.

78. Bonnard A, Zamakhshary M, de Silva N, et al. Non-operative management of gastroschisis: a case-matched study. Pediatr Surg Int 2008;24:767–71.

79. Riboh J, Abrajano CT, Garber K, et al. Outcomes of sutureless gastroschisis closure. J Pediatr Surg 2009;44:1947–51.

80. Orion KC, Krein M, Liao J, et al. Outcomes of plastic closure in gastroschisis. Surgery 2011;150(2):177–85.

81. Hassan SF, Pimpalwar A. Primary suture-less closure of gastroschisis using negative pressure dressing (wound vacuum). Eur J Pediatr Surg 2011;21:287–91.

82. Abdullah F, Arnold MA, Nabaweesi R, et al. Gastroschisis in the United States 1988-2003: analysis and risk categorization of 4344 patients. J Perinatol 2007; 27:50–5.

83. Arnold MA, Chang DC, Nabaweesi R, et al. Development and validation of a risk stratification index to predict death in gastroschisis. J Pediatr Surg 2007;42: 950–5 [discussion: 5–6].

84. Arnold MA, Chang DC, Nabaweesi R, et al. Risk stratification of 4344 patients with gastroschisis into simple and complex categories. J Pediatr Surg 2007;42: 1520–5.

85. Fleet MS, de la Hunt MN. Intestinal atresia with gastroschisis: a selective approach to management. J Pediatr Surg 2000;35:1323–5.

86. Snyder CL, Miller KA, Sharp RJ, et al. Management of intestinal atresia in patients with gastroschisis. J Pediatr Surg 2001;36:1542–5.

87. Hill SJ, Durham MM. Management of cryptorchidism and gastroschisis. J Pediatr Surg 2011;46:1798–803.

88. Davies BW, Stringer MD. The survivors of gastroschisis. Arch Dis Child 1997;77: 158–60.

Necrotizing Enterocolitis

Kathleen M. Dominguez, MD, R. Lawrence Moss, MD*

KEYWORDS

- Necrotizing enterocolitis • Prematurity • Pneumatosis intestinalis
- Peritoneal drainage • Short gut syndrome • Intestinal failure
- Neurodevelopmental outcomes

KEY POINTS

- Necrotizing enterocolitis (NEC) is a serious cause of morbidity and mortality in premature infants.
- Despite improvements in neonatal care, the incidence of NEC has increased and mortality remains unchanged.
- The pathogenesis of NEC is multifactorial, but is believed to include factors such as intestinal and immunologic immaturity, ischemia, hypoxia, genetic predisposition, and feeding practices.
- Neonates who require surgical treatment of NEC fare worse in terms of mortality, neurodevelopmental outcomes, and gastrointestinal morbidity.

INTRODUCTION

Necrotizing enterocolitis (NEC) is primarily a disease of premature infants, and remains a leading cause of death in the neonatal intensive care unit (NICU). As neonatal care has advanced over the last 30 years, the incidence of NEC has increased and mortality has remained unchanged. Despite early, aggressive treatment, the progression of bowel necrosis can lead to sepsis and death. Survivors, particularly those who require surgery, suffer significant morbidity in terms of gastrointestinal (GI) disease and poor neurodevelopmental outcomes. Despite decades of rigorous research, few advances have been made in the care of infants once NEC has been established; prevention of this often fatal disease is likely to have the greatest overall impact on morbidity and mortality.

EPIDEMIOLOGY

NEC is the most common GI emergency affecting premature infants, particularly those infants classified as very low birth weight (VLBW, <1500 g) or extremely low birth weight

Department of Surgery, Nationwide Children's Hospital, The Ohio State University College of Medicine, 700 Children's Drive, Columbus, OH 43205, USA
* Corresponding author.
E-mail address: larry.moss@nationwidechildrens.org

Clin Perinatol 39 (2012) 387–401
doi:10.1016/j.clp.2012.04.011
0095-5108/12/$ – see front matter © 2012 Elsevier Inc. All rights reserved.

perinatology.theclinics.com

(ELBW, <1000 g)[1–3] The overall incidence of NEC is approximately 1 in 1000 live births,[3–5] but in infants less than 1500 g, the incidence increases to between 3% and 10%.[6–9] The incidence shows a clear, inverse relationship with birth weight and gestational age.[4,6,10] The incidence of NEC has increased in recent years, as a result of advances in neonatal intensive care, which allow younger, sicker infants (the population most at risk for NEC) to survive.[11,12] Black infants, and in particular black males, are significantly more likely to develop NEC,[3,6] even when correcting for birth weight.[2,4,8,13]

Mortality from the disease, overall ranging from 15% to 30%, is higher in those with lower birth weight and younger gestational age, and male infants.[2,10,14] In addition, black males have a higher rate of mortality associated with NEC.[2] A particularly severe form of NEC, termed NEC totalis or fulminant NEC, in which the entire intestine is affected, has a mortality of more than 90%.[15–17] These infants tend to have lower birth weight and earlier gestational age than infants affected with less severe NEC.[16]

Most NEC cases occur in premature infants, with an incidence of approximately 0.5 per 1000 in term or near-term live births.[18,19] Full-term infants who develop NEC typically have specific risk factors, including congenital heart disease, sepsis, or hypotension.[18,20,21] What seems to be the common feature of these predisposing conditions is reduced mesenteric perfusion.[22–24] The mortality for term infants with NEC seems to be similar to that seen in premature infants with NEC.[1,8]

Spontaneous intestinal perforation (also called isolated or focal intestinal perforation) is defined as bowel perforation without other evidence of NEC on physical or radiographic examination. Much like classic NEC, this disease process occurs in VLBW and ELBW infants. An association has been found with indomethacin and with glucocorticoid exposure.[25] This process typically occurs within a few days after birth, and is not associated with the onset of feeding.[24] Unlike classic NEC, there is not significant intestinal inflammation, and systemic markers of inflammation, such as serum cytokines, are low.[26] Typical radiographic findings are pneumoperitoneum in the absence of pneumatosis.[27] Controversy exists as to whether this finding is a subset of NEC or a distinct clinical entity. The preoperative differentiation between classic NEC and spontaneous intestinal perforation is difficult, with even experienced surgeons often wrong in their preoperative diagnosis.[28]

Medical management is sufficient for most patients with NEC, but 20% to 40% develop severe enough disease to require surgical intervention.[3,9] Outcomes in patients who require surgical intervention are significantly worse than those seen in patients who improve with medical management alone. Mortality for surgical NEC is roughly 50%, and has not significantly changed over the past 30 years.[3,9,14] In addition, infants who survive are more likely to have long-term complications such as neurodevelopmental delay, growth delay, and chronic GI problems.[9]

In addition to the medical implications for babies who develop NEC, there is also an enormous societal economic burden because of the disease. The estimated annual cost for caring with infants affected by NEC in the United States is between $500 million and $1 billion.[26] Bisquera and colleagues[29] performed a case-control analysis evaluating the impact of NEC on hospital length of stay and hospital charges in VLBW infants. These investigators found that, on average, infants with medically treated NEC had an NICU length of stay exceeding controls by 22 days, and infants with surgically treated NEC had a length of stay exceeding controls by 60 days. Hospital costs were also substantially higher than that seen for controls, averaging $73,700 higher for medically treated infants and $186,200 higher for surgically treated infants. These estimates do not include costs associated with long-term morbidity seen in NEC survivors, including short bowel syndrome (SBS), parenteral nutrition (PN)-associated liver disease, and neurodevelopmental delay. The economic burden of these outcomes is substantial, but has not been quantified.

PATHOGENESIS
Intrinsic Factors

The pathogenesis of NEC is not clearly defined, but is likely multifactorial. NEC is a severe inflammatory disorder, which can involve any portion of the GI tract, but most typically involves the ileum and proximal colon.[30,31] Intestinal involvement can be patchy, focal, or diffuse.[31] NEC is believed to represent an inappropriate or over-exuberant inflammatory response to some type of insult. The nature of the insult is not well defined, and may vary between infants. It may be a global ischemic insult related to congenital heart disease or sepsis, an infectious insult from bacteria, or an insult related to formula feeding. This initial insult results in disruption of the intestinal epithelium, bacterial translocation, and an exaggerated immune response by immature intestinal epithelial cells.[32] Classic histologic findings include inflammation, bacterial overgrowth, and coagulation necrosis, and are seen in nearly all affected infants.[30,33] As the disease progresses, the injury progresses to full-thickness intestinal wall, after which perforation can occur.

The neonatal intestinal tract is immature in many ways, and this seems to predispose premature infants to intestinal injury. Abnormalities in motility, digestion, circulatory regulation, barrier function, and immune defense are all present. Motility normally develops during the third trimester of pregnancy.[34] In premature infants, decreased motility leads to slowed transit of intestinal contents and increased bacterial load, and exposure of the intestinal epithelium to potentially noxious substances.[4,35,36] Digestion and absorption are also decreased and may further exacerbate this problem.[12,37,38] These factors likely also contribute to abnormal microbial colonization of the intestine in premature infants.

The intestinal epithelium plays a key role in protection against potential pathogens and acts as both a physical and biochemical barrier. In premature infants, tight junctions, which function to zipper together the intestinal epithelia, are incompletely developed, allowing for increased permeability.[12,32,35,39] The mucin layer acts not only as a physical barrier but also aids in aggregation and removal of adherent bacteria, as well as in trapping enzymes near the epithelial surface to enhance digestion. In premature infants, the composition and volume of this layer is less mature and, hence, less effective, allowing for increased bacterial adherence and permeability.[12,32]

Immunologic function of the neonatal intestinal tract is also immature, which plays an important role in the pathogenesis of NEC. This immaturity, which involves many facets of the immune system, from antigen processing and presentation to production of antibacterial compounds, leads to abnormal microbial colonization.[21,39] Secretory IgA, which functions to bind luminal bacteria, is not produced until several weeks postnatally.[12] In addition, many premature infants receive antibiotics, and this likely has an influence on bacterial colonization.[20,36] Normally, the flora that populate the intestinal tract act to modulate the immune system and play an important role in maintaining the intestinal barrier; as the composition of the flora changes, the modulation of the immune response is lost.[25] A local insult, which in a more mature infant would be contained by the local immune system in the gut, can quickly lead to bacterial translocation and an exuberant systemic inflammatory response in a premature infant.

Ischemia and hypoxia also seem to be important in the pathogenesis of NEC. In the microvasculature of the intestine there is a fine balance between vasodilation and vasoconstriction. Nitric oxide (NO) is normally present at low levels and acts as a local vasodilator, maintaining low systemic vascular resistance. NO is produced from argi-nine by NO synthase (NOS); there are 3 isoforms of NOS: endothelial NOS (eNOS), neuronal NOS (nNOS), and inducible NOS (iNOS). Although eNOS and nNOS produce NO at constitutively low levels, inflammation can cause sustained upregulation of iNOS, leading to a million-fold increase in NO production.[40] In higher concentrations NO has been shown to cause direct epithelial injury and apoptosis.[11,12,22,25,39,40] In addition, overproduction of NO has been implicated in impaired mucosal healing after an initial insult. This situation seems to lead to a sustained defect in the barrier function and prolonged activation of the inflammatory cascade.[12,40] Endothelin 1 (ET-1) is the primary mediator of vasoconstriction in the newborn intestinal circulation[22,41,42]; ET-1 is a potent vasoconstrictor, and because of a unique interaction with its receptor, can induce sustained ischemia for hours.[33] Production of ET-1 is upregulated by a wide range of stimuli, including hypoxia and inflammatory cytokines.[22,33] In pathologic states, the balance between NO and ET-1 is upset and vasoconstriction occurs, leading to intestinal ischemia and tissue injury.[41,42]

Several key mediators have been identified in the pathogenesis of NEC. Three of these mediators are lipopolysaccharide (LPS), tumor necrosis factor α (TNF-α), and platelet activating factor (PAF). LPS is the endotoxin component of gram-negative bacteria and acts as an important inflammatory mediator. LPS acts to impair intestinal barrier function and promotes the release of other inflammatory mediators, such as NO and interferon γ, which have a direct cytotoxic effect on intestinal epithelial cells.[25,39,43] LPS is used in animal models to experimentally induce NEC.[44] TNF-α is an inflammatory cytokine that has been found to be present in increased levels in neonates with NEC, and administration of TNF-α has also been found to lead to increased production of PAF.[45] PAF is an endogenous inflammatory mediator, the effects of which are compounded by LPS[43] and by ET-1.[33,46] PAF has also been shown to cause bowel injury and apoptosis through the formation of oxygen-derived free radicals,[43,45,46] and is seen at higher circulating levels in patients with NEC.[33,47]

Premature infants are prone to abnormal bacterial colonization for many reasons. Alterations in peristalsis, digestion, absorption, and immune function have already been discussed. In addition, premature infants are colonized by fewer bacterial strains than term neonates,[20,26] and are more likely to be colonized by pathogenic bacteria,[32] such as *Klebsiella, Enterobacter* and *Clostridiums* species.[8] Although no specific species of bacteria has been implicated in the pathogenesis of NEC, it seems that this alteration in gut flora predisposes to a breach of the immature intestinal barrier and the resulting inflammatory cascade that defines NEC.

Extrinsic Factors

Feeding practices have long been implicated in the development of NEC. This theory has been difficult to clearly elucidate, because feeding practices have varied signifi-cantly with time, as well as from NICU to NICU. Several case-control and retrospective studies have reported that feeding or increasing feeds too rapidly seems to increase the risk of NEC[48,49]; however, Cochrane systematic reviews[50–53] examining feeding practices including delayed introduction of enteral feeds and slow advancement of enteral feed volumes have failed to show a significant association. Similarly, a Cochrane review[50] comparing trophic feeding with no feeding or advancing feeding practices showed no consistent results in terms of incidence of NEC, and hence no clear benefit to either practice regarding NEC. Standardized feeding protocols or feeding guidelines, which typically involve initiation of feeding based on gestational age of the infant and slow gradual advancement of both volumes and concentration, have been shown to have a lower incidence of NEC compared with nonstandardized initiation of feeds.[27,54,55] In addition, the use of feeding guidelines has been shown to improve growth, reduce the length of stay, and lower hospital costs.[27]

Human breast milk is well known to have antimicrobial and antiinflammatory properties.[27,45] Breast milk would be expected to have a protective effect against the development of NEC, but this has been difficult to study clinically because of lack of standardized definitions of what is considered human breast milk. Variations in human breast milk feeding practices include maternal versus donor breast milk, use of fortification and type of fortifier, and whether infants are fed only breast milk or supplemented with formula. Meta-analyses have suggested that the use of human milk reduces the incidence of NEC,[56,57] and that fortification of milk does not increase the incidence of NEC.[58] A recent prospective, randomized trial comparing the exclusive use of human breast milk with bovine milk-based products found that the incidence of NEC was 77% lower in infants exclusively fed human breast milk and that the incidence of NEC requiring surgical intervention was also significantly lower.[59]

Gastric pH seems to play a role in the development of NEC, presumably because of an alteration in the bacterial flora of the intestinal tract. Accordingly, infants who are treated with histamine 2 blockers have an increased incidence of NEC.[6] It remains unclear whether this is a causative association or a marker of general illness in patients thus already at increased risk of developing NEC. Similarly, infants with anemia seem to be at increased risk of NEC, and a temporal association of the onset on NEC is seen after transfusions of red blood cells.[60] Again, it is unclear whether the anemia and resultant transfusions are a cause of NEC or a marker of more severely ill infants at risk for the development of the disease.

Clinical presentation

NEC can vary widely in its presentation, from a slow, indolent course, to a rapidly progressive illness resulting in death in just a few hours.[61,62] Clinical signs of NEC are often nonspecific and include apnea, bradycardia, temperature instability, lethargy, mottling, and increase in need for ventilatory support.[63] Infants may show feeding intolerance (increased residuals or emesis), abdominal distension/increased girth, bloody stools, discoloration of the abdominal wall, or a palpable mass.[63]

Laboratory findings include nonspecific indicators of inflammation such as leukocytosis and bandemia. Thrombocytopenia is also common, and is a poor prognostic indicator when the decrease in platelets is rapid. Metabolic acidosis and increased C-reactive protein (CRP) levels are also common findings. Multiple studies have attempted to find unique biochemical markers for NEC or markers of disease severity in those affected, but thus far, this has not been successful. CRP can be useful in monitoring the course of the disease. Ordinarily, this marker normalizes as inflammation subsides; a persistent increase can be suggestive of a complication such as abscess, stricture, or fistula.

The hallmark radiographic finding of NEC is pneumatosis intestinalis (**Fig. 1A**). This condition may be linear or cystic, and is the most common radiographic finding associated with NEC. More severe disease may have portal venous gas[64] (see **Fig. 1A**); this finding is a poor prognostic indicator. Pneumoperitoneum indicates full-thickness intestinal injury with perforation (see **Fig. 1B**). Other less specific findings that may be seen in NEC include dilated loops of bowel with or without air fluid levels, thickened bowel wall, a paucity of gas (gasless abdomen), or dilated loops of bowel that are unaltered on repeat examinations (fixed loops). Radiographs should include both a supine and dependent view (cross-table lateral or left lateral decubitus) to fully evaluate for pneumoperitoneum.

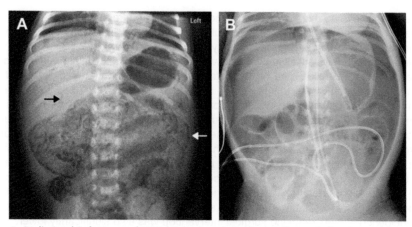

Fig. 1. Radiographic features of NEC. (*A*) Supine abdominal radiograph showing pneumatosis intestinalis (*white arrow*) and portal venous gas (*black arrow*). (*B*) Supine abdominal radiograph showing pneumoperitoneum, a sign of advanced NEC and indication for surgical intervention.

The role of ultrasonography in the evaluation of NEC is not yet clear. This modality can be used to assess bowel wall viability (using color Doppler), as well as assess bowel wall thickness, peristalsis, fluid collections with presence of particulate debris, pneumatosis, or portal venous gas, and may be useful in cases in which radiographs do not match the clinical picture.[65] Further studies are needed to define the role of ultrasonography in the evaluation of NEC. Other modalities, such as computed tomography or magnetic resonance imaging, do not have a role in the evaluation of NEC.

A staging system for NEC was first proposed by Bell in 1978.[66] This system, which has undergone modification since, uses a combination of historical factors, systemic manifestations, GI manifestations, and radiographic manifestations, to assign a stage, which can then be used to determine treatment, and is also useful for categorizing the severity of disease for research purposes (**Table 1**).

DIFFERENTIAL DIAGNOSIS

In ill neonates, a septic ileus can present similarly to NEC, with a distended abdomen, increased residuals and clinical signs of sepsis. In addition, NEC may not always have classic radiographic or other clinical findings. Sometimes these 2 entities can be differentiated only by monitoring the course of the disease over time. For this reason, it is important to consider and treat potential causes of sepsis. Careful abdominal examination and radiographs are key in the evaluation of an infant with abdominal distension, and can help differentiate between NEC, intestinal atresia, Hirschsprung disease, volvulus, and meconium disease.[25]

Neonates who are not acutely ill may also show some of the clinical signs seen in NEC. A distended abdomen or increased residuals may be seen with meconium disease of prematurity or a nonspecific feeding intolerance. Bloody stools can be seen with anal fissure or milk protein allergy.

TREATMENT

Most patients affected by NEC can be managed medically. When clinical, laboratory, and radiographic findings are suspicious for NEC, initial management should include bowel rest; abdominal decompression with a gastric tube; cultures of the blood, urine,

Table 1
Modified Bell criteria for staging NEC

Stage	Systemic Criteria	Abdominal Criteria	Radiographic Criteria
1a: suspected NEC	Temperature instability, apnea, bradycardia	Increased pregavage residuals, mild abdominal distension, occult blood in stool	Normal or intestinal dilatation, mild ileus
1b: suspected NEC	Same as above	Grossly bloody stool	Same as above
2a: definite NEC; mildly ill	Same as above	Same as stage 1 plus lack of bowel sounds, possible abdominal tenderness	Ileus, pneumatosis intestinalis
2b: definite NEC; moderately ill	Same as stage 1 plus mild metabolic acidosis, mild thrombocytopenia	Same as above plus peritonitis, definite abdominal tenderness, possible cellulitis, right lower quadrant mass	Same as above plus possible portal venous gas
3a: advanced NEC; severely ill, intact bowel	Same as stage 2b plus hypotension, severe apnea, combined respiratory and metabolic acidosis, disseminated intravascular coagulation, and neutropenia	Same as above with marked tenderness and abdominal distension	Same as above plus ascites
3b: advanced NEC; severely ill, perforated bowel	Same as stage 3a	Same as stage 3a	Pneumoperitoneum

and sputum; and administration of broad spectrum antibiotics. Intravenous fluid resuscitation and PN are initiated. Depending on the clinical condition, additional supportive care may be necessary, including increased ventilator support, support of blood pressure with pressors, or blood transfusions. Serial abdominal examinations and abdominal radiographs should be performed and often dictate when surgical management is indicated. Expectant medical management remains appropriate if the patient's condition is stable or improving. The duration of antibiotic treatment is not clear and has not been well studied; typical practices are 7 to 14 days.

The only absolute indication for surgery is frank bowel perforation, as indicated by pneumoperitoneum on abdominal films, or the presence of stool or bile on paracentesis.[9,15] A relative indication is clinical deterioration despite maximal medical therapy. In the past, the presence of portal venous gas was often used as an indication for operative intervention. Although this finding does infer a poor prognosis, retrospective studies have had conflicting results. One study reported that 47% of infants with this finding on plain abdominal radiograph survived without an operation,[9] whereas another reported that 93% of infants with portal venous gas have full-thickness bowel necrosis at the time of surgery.[15] Other relative indications for surgery include fixed loops on abdominal radiograph, erythema of the abdominal wall, and a palpable abdominal mass. These indications must be taken in context with the overall clinical condition of the patient, because they are neither sensitive nor specific.

When surgical intervention is performed, the 2 primary means of treatment are laparotomy and primary peritoneal drainage (PPD). Traditionally, surgical management of NEC consisted of laparotomy with resection of clearly ischemic bowel and the creation of ostomies (**Fig. 2**). In 1977, placement of a peritoneal drain was described by Ein and colleagues.[67] The operation was initially proposed for patients considered too unstable for laparotomy, and was intended to be used only as a temporizing measure until definitive treatment could be performed. Over time, PPD has become an accepted alternative to laparotomy and is used as a definitive treatment in many cases, although controversy exists as to whether the laparotomy or PPD approach is superior. Three prospective studies have been conducted to compare laparotomy with PPD; all have failed to show clear superiority of either method. The initial study, a prospective observational cohort study, was performed with data from 16 centers through the National Institute of Child Health and Human Development Neonatal Research Network. Initial findings suggested that laparotomy had a decreased risk of adverse outcomes; however, the treatment groups were not similar. When adjustments were made to reflect differences between the treatment groups, there was no longer evidence of a reduction in adverse outcomes with laparotomy.[14]

Two subsequent randomized trials have compared laparotomy with PPD in perforated NEC. The Necrotizing Enterocolitis Study Towards Evidence-based Pediatric Surgery trial randomized 117 infants of less than 1500 g to either PPD or laparotomy. No difference in mortality at 90 days was found. Secondary outcomes, such as length of hospitalization and dependence on PN at 90 days, were also similar between the 2 groups.[68] The Necrotizing Enterocolitis trial compared PPD and laparotomy in infants of less than 1000 g worldwide. The main outcome was mortality at 1 and 6 months, and no significant difference was found between the 2 groups. However, a large percentage of infants in the PPD group (74%) underwent delayed laparotomy, and only 11% of patients survived with PPD alone.[69]

POSTOPERATIVE CARE AND SHORT-TERM OUTCOMES

Infants who require surgical treatment of NEC require ongoing physiologic support postoperatively. This support includes fluid resuscitation, and pressor and ventilator support as necessary. Antibiotics are typically continued for 7 to 14 days, and gastric decompression is continued until there is evidence of bowel function. PN is maintained until enteral feeding is appropriate. Once bowel function returns, feedings are slowly

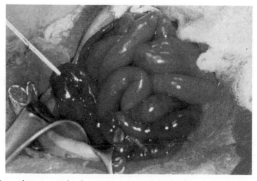

Fig. 2. Intraoperative photograph showing necrotic bowel and adjacent healthy bowel.

advanced, with careful attention to stoma output. Patients who do not have sufficient small bowel remaining to absorb full enteral nutrition are maintained on long-term PN. Typically, patients are able to be weaned off PN over several months. For those patients with insufficient intestinal length or function, surgical options such as intestinal lengthening procedures or transplantation may be considered once the child is older.

Approximately 5% of NEC cases recur; these patients can usually be managed non-operatively.[35,70] Disease can recur at the initial site, or anywhere along the GI tract. Recurrent NEC is more common in patients with underlying disease, such as congenital heart disease. The mortality for recurrent NEC is similar to that for primary NEC.[70]

Complications related to the stoma are seen in at least half of patients who survive; these include retraction, prolapse, hernia, and wound infection.[71,72] Although many techniques for ostomy creation exist, none has been shown to be superior in terms of function or complications. Patients with proximal ostomies can have significant issues with fluid losses and resulting electrolyte imbalances, resulting in failure to gain weight, dehydration, and skin breakdown.

In patients who have had laparotomy and stoma creation, consideration must be given to the timing of stoma takedown. There is variation in practice between surgeons, with most waiting at least 1 month and some as many as 4 months after the initial operation. Timing of stoma takedown may also be based on patient weight (typically at least 2000 g) and overall medical condition, including adequate nutrition and growth.[17]

An additional complication that can be seen in patients who have recovered from NEC is stricture. Stricture can occur in both patients who are medically managed and those undergoing surgery and is seen in 10% to 40% of patients.[28,71] Most often, these strictures occur in the left colon.[71,73] There does not seem to be any difference between choice of surgical technique and stricture formation, with an equal incidence seen in patients undergoing PPD and laparotomy.[72]

PROGNOSIS/LONG-TERM OUTCOMES

Mortality from NEC remains high, averaging 10% to 50%, despite the many advances made in the care of premature infants.[28] For those infants who do survive, long-term difficulties with GI morbidity and poor neurodevelopmental outcome are a persistent issue.

The most common long-term GI complication is SBS. SBS is defined as inadequate intestine to absorb nutrients for growth.[73] Approximately one-fourth of survivors of NEC requiring surgical treatment are affected, with those having undergone more extensive bowel resection at the greatest risk.[15,74] Multiple studies have shown that the ability to wean from PN correlates with the length of residual intestine.[75] However, intestinal length is not the only determinant of adequate GI function, because SBS is also seen in patients who have not had resection (those who underwent PPD), or sometimes in patients with medically managed NEC. Despite normal intestinal length, the absorptive capacity of the intestine may be poor in areas that were involved in the disease process. The likelihood of SBS is also influenced by the portion of the intestine that is affected or resected; certain portions of the intestine have a greater capacity to undergo adaptation, with the ileum being the most adaptive. As a result, patients with jejunal disease tend to fare better long-term than patients who require extensive resection of the ileum. Although conventional wisdom indicated that those with an intact ileocecal valve fare better, the data are mixed and the overall outcome seems to be more influenced by intestinal length and functionality.[73] Other common GI issues seen in patients with NEC include constipation, encopresis, gastroesophageal reflux disease, and bowel obstruction.[28,76]

For those infants dependent on long-term PN, liver disease is a serious problem. Since the development of PN, mortality secondary to dehydration and malnutrition has essentially been eliminated; however, patients on long-term PN commonly develop serious hepatic dysfunction, a condition known as PN-associated liver disease (PNALD). PNALD is characterized by steatosis, cholestasis, and inflammatory changes. Over time, PNALD can progress to fibrosis and cirrhosis: 40% to 60% of pediatric patients receiving prolonged PN develop PNALD.[74,77] Patients who develop PNALD have an increased mortality of 80% to 90%.[78] Other complications associated with prolonged use of PN include recurrent central venous catheter sepsis and poor bone mineralization. Complications are correlated to duration of PN.[75]

Even for patients without SBS, growth may be affected. When compared with patients without NEC and patients with medically managed NEC, patients with surgically managed NEC were significantly more likely to have substantial growth delay.[79]

Neurologic outcomes are a major problem in survivors of NEC, a realization that Stevenson was among the first to describe in 1980.[80] Although patients with medically managed NEC are likely to be similar to matched controls in terms of growth and development, survivors of surgically treated NEC are nearly twice as likely to have neurodevelopmental impairment, and developmental delay is seen in approximately 50% of patients.[28,76,79] Dysfunction is often shown in vision, auditory, speech, motor, and intellectual delays, as well as problems with interpersonal and social skills.[28,76,79] A prospective observational cohort study performed by Blakely and colleagues[28] suggests that patients treated with PPD fare worse in terms of neurodevelopmental outcomes when compared with patients treated with laparotomy. No firm conclusions could be drawn because of significant differences between the treatment groups; however, this finding does raise concerns, and underscores the need for further research.

PREVENTION

Given that surgical strategies do not seem to have a major effect on morbidity and mortality related to NEC, prevention seems to have the greatest potential for avoiding adverse outcomes. Currently proven strategies for prevention include the use of human breast milk and standardized feeding protocols, as previously discussed. These 2 programs are additive and likely even synergistic in their effect on reducing the incidence of NEC; it has been estimated that together, these 2 programs can decrease the incidence of NEC by half.[27]

Probiotics also seem to have promise, and have been described as living microorganisms that are ingested with the intention of colonizing and replicating within the intestinal tract.[8] The mechanisms of probiotics action seem to be multifactorial; at least in part, their actions can be attributed to modulation of the immune response, strengthening of the intestinal barrier, and production of antibacterial substances.[81] Although exact ingredients vary, these supplements contain potentially beneficial bacteria and yeast, most commonly *Lactobacillus*, *Bifidobacterium*, and *Streptococcus*.[32,35,81] Probiotics may aid in normalizing the colonization of the neonatal gut and in improving intestinal function. A Cochrane review[82] of probiotic use identified a reduced incidence of NEC in neonates treated with probiotics as well as a decrease in the mortality. Although these results are encouraging, the specifications are not known regarding strain selection, dose, and duration of supplementation, age to begin therapy, or long-term implications of probiotic use. Although it did not seem increased in the meta-analysis, the risk of sepsis secondary to the probiotic organism is of particular concern in neonates. Isolated reports of sepsis secondary to the use of *Lactobacillus* species in both adult and pediatric patients have been reported,[21] and a recent multicenter trial of probiotics noted a trend toward a higher incidence of sepsis in infants receiving probiotics, particularly those with a birth weight less than 750 g.[20] Continued research is needed to determine the safety and efficacy of probiotic usage for the prevention of NEC.

FUTURE DIRECTIONS

Epidermal growth factor (EGF) is a peptide secreted into the intestinal lumen, and is active in a variety of biologic responses from cell replication/movement to cell survival.[83] EGF has been shown to support maintenance of the intestinal barrier and is active in downregulation of inflammatory cytokines.[35] Heparin-binding EGF (HB-EGF) is a member of this family of growth factors, and is found in amniotic fluid and human breast milk.[27] In animal models of NEC, administration of HB-EGF has been shown to reduce the incidence of bowel injury by half and more than double survival.[84–86] Animals with overexpression of HB-EGF have decreased susceptibility to NEC[87]; conversely, animals with a deletion of the HB-EGF gene have increased susceptibility.[44,88] These effects seem to be at least in part a result of HB-EGF cytoprotective effects, functioning to protect intestinal stem cells from injury.[44] Clinical trials testing HB-EGF treatment in the prevention of NEC are soon to be under way.

SUMMARY

NEC is a significant cause of morbidity and mortality in neonates; despite several decades of research, little headway has been made in reducing the impact of this disease. The only consistently shown risk factor is prematurity, and clinical parameters do not seem to be able to predict which infants are likely to develop NEC. Most of the morbidity and mortality from the disease is seen in patients who require surgical intervention. The choice of operation does not seem to influence the outcome. Therefore, preventative strategies are likely to have the greatest impact in positively influencing outcomes.

REFERENCES

1. Lambert DK, Christensen RD, Henry E, et al. Necrotizing enterocolitis in term neonates: data from a multihospital health-care system. J Perinatol 2007;27(7): 437–43.
2. Holman RC, Stoll BJ, Clarke MJ, et al. The epidemiology of necrotizing enterocolitis infant mortality in the United States. Am J Public Health 1997;87(12):2026–31.
3. Holman RC, Stoll BJ, Curns AT, et al. Necrotising enterocolitis hospitalisations among neonates in the United States. Paediatr Perinat Epidemiol 2006;20(6): 498–506.
4. Llanos AR, Moss ME, Pinzon MC, et al. Epidemiology of neonatal necrotising enterocolitis: a population-based study. Paediatr Perinat Epidemiol 2002;16(4):342–9.
5. Holman RC, Stehr-Green JK, Zelasky MT. Necrotizing enterocolitis mortality in the United States, 1979-85. Am J Public Health 1989;79(8):987–9.
6. Guillet R, Stoll BJ, Cotten CM, et al. Association of H2-blocker therapy and higher incidence of necrotizing enterocolitis in very low birth weight infants. Pediatrics 2006;117(2):e137–42.
7. Sankaran K, Puckett B, Lee DS, et al. Variations in incidence of necrotizing enterocolitis in Canadian neonatal intensive care units. J Pediatr Gastroenterol Nutr 2004;39(4):366–72.
8. Srinivasan PS, Brandler MD, D'Souza A. Necrotizing enterocolitis. Clin Perinatol 2008;35(1):251–72, x.

9. Blakely ML, Gupta H, Lally KP. Surgical management of necrotizing enterocolitis and isolated intestinal perforation in premature neonates. Semin Perinatol 2008; 32(2):122–6.

10. Fitzgibbons SC, Ching Y, Yu D, et al. Mortality of necrotizing enterocolitis expressed by birth weight categories. J Pediatr Surg 2009;44(6):1072–5 [discussion: 1075–6].

11. Petrosyan M, Guner YS, Williams M, et al. Current concepts regarding the pathogenesis of necrotizing enterocolitis. Pediatr Surg Int 2009;25(4):309–18.

12. Ford HR. Mechanism of nitric oxide-mediated intestinal barrier failure: insight into the pathogenesis of necrotizing enterocolitis. J Pediatr Surg 2006;41(2):294–9.

13. Uauy RD, Fanaroff AA, Korones SB, et al. Necrotizing enterocolitis in very low birth weight infants: biodemographic and clinical correlates. National Institute of Child Health and Human Development Neonatal Research Network. J Pediatr 1991;119(4):630–8.

14. Blakely ML, Lally KP, McDonald S, et al. Postoperative outcomes of extremely low birth-weight infants with necrotizing enterocolitis or isolated intestinal perforation: a prospective cohort study by the NICHD Neonatal Research Network. Ann Surg 2005;241(6):984–9 [discussion: 989–94].

15. Henry MC, Lawrence Moss R. Surgical therapy for necrotizing enterocolitis: bringing evidence to the bedside. Semin Pediatr Surg 2005;14(3):181–90.

16. Lambert DK, Christensen RD, Baer VL, et al. Fulminant necrotizing enterocolitis in a multihospital healthcare system. J Perinatol 2012;32(3):194–8.

17. Albanese CT, Rowe MI. Necrotizing enterocolitis. Semin Pediatr Surg 1995;4(4): 200–6.

18. Bolisetty S, Lui K, Oei J, et al. A regional study of underlying congenital diseases in term neonates with necrotizing enterocolitis. Acta Paediatr 2000;89(10):1226–30.

19. Obladen M. Necrotizing enterocolitis–150 years of fruitless search for the cause. Neonatology 2009;96(4):203–10.

20. Murgas Torrazza R, Neu J. The developing intestinal microbiome and its relationship to health and disease in the neonate. J Perinatol 2011;31(Suppl 1):S29–34.

21. Hunter CJ, Upperman JS, Ford HR, et al. Understanding the susceptibility of the premature infant to necrotizing enterocolitis (NEC). Pediatr Res 2008;63(2):117–23.

22. Nankervis CA, Giannone PJ, Reber KM. The neonatal intestinal vasculature: contributing factors to necrotizing enterocolitis. Semin Perinatol 2008;32(2): 83–91.

23. McElhinney DB, Hedrick HL, Bush DM, et al. Necrotizing enterocolitis in neonates with congenital heart disease: risk factors and outcomes. Pediatrics 2000;106(5):1080–7.

24. Young CM, Kingma SD, Neu J. Ischemia-reperfusion and neonatal intestinal injury. J Pediatr 2011;158(Suppl 2):e25–8.

25. Berman L, Moss RL. Necrotizing enterocolitis: an update. Semin Fetal Neonatal Med 2011;16(3):145–50.

26. Neu J, Walker WA. Necrotizing enterocolitis. N Engl J Med 2011;364(3):255–64.

27. Christensen RD, Gordon PV, Besner GE. Can we cut the incidence of necrotizing enterocolitis in half–today? Fetal Pediatr Pathol 2010;29(4):185–98.

28. Blakely ML, Tyson JE, Lally KP, et al. Laparotomy versus peritoneal drainage for necrotizing enterocolitis or isolated intestinal perforation in extremely low birth weight infants: outcomes through 18 months adjusted age. Pediatrics 2006; 117(4):e680–7.

29. Bisquera JA, Cooper TR, Berseth CL. Impact of necrotizing enterocolitis on length of stay and hospital charges in very low birth weight infants. Pediatrics 2002;109(3):423–8.

30. Ballance WA, Dahms BB, Shenker N, et al. Pathology of neonatal necrotizing enterocolitis: a ten-year experience. J Pediatr 1990;117(1 Pt 2):S6–13.
31. Zhang Y, Ortega G, Camp M, et al. Necrotizing enterocolitis requiring surgery: outcomes by intestinal location of disease in 4371 infants. J Pediatr Surg 2011; 46(8):1475–81.
32. Lin PW, Nasr TR, Stoll BJ. Necrotizing enterocolitis: recent scientific advances in pathophysiology and prevention. Semin Perinatol 2008;32(2):70–82.
33. Nowicki PT, Caniano DA, Hammond S, et al. Endothelial nitric oxide synthase in human intestine resected for necrotizing enterocolitis. J Pediatr 2007;150(1):40–5.
34. Sanderson IR. The physicochemical environment of the neonatal intestine. Am J Clin Nutr 1999;69(5):1028S–34S.
35. Henry MC, Moss RL. Necrotizing enterocolitis. Annu Rev Med 2009;60:111–24.
36. Indrio F, Neu J. The intestinal microbiome of infants and the use of probiotics. Curr Opin Pediatr 2011;23(2):145–50.
37. Lebenthal A, Lebenthal E. The ontogeny of the small intestinal epithelium. JPEN J Parenter Enteral Nutr 1999;23(Suppl 5):S3–6.
38. Di Lorenzo M, Bass J, Krantis A. An intraluminal model of necrotizing enterocolitis in the developing neonatal piglet. J Pediatr Surg 1995;30(8):1138–42.
39. Emami CN, Petrosyan M, Giuliani S, et al. Role of the host defense system and intestinal microbial flora in the pathogenesis of necrotizing enterocolitis. Surg Infect (Larchmt) 2009;10(5):407–17.
40. Chokshi NK, Guner YS, Hunter CJ, et al. The role of nitric oxide in intestinal epithelial injury and restitution in neonatal necrotizing enterocolitis. Semin Perinatol 2008;32(2):92–9.
41. Nowicki PT. Ischemia and necrotizing enterocolitis: where, when, and how. Semin Pediatr Surg 2005;14(3):152–8.
42. Nowicki PT, Dunaway DJ, Nankervis CA, et al. Endothelin-1 in human intestine resected for necrotizing enterocolitis. J Pediatr 2005;146(6):805–10.
43. Anand RJ, Leaphart CL, Mollen KP, et al. The role of the intestinal barrier in the pathogenesis of necrotizing enterocolitis. Shock 2007;27(2):124–33.
44. Chen CL, Yu X, James IO, et al. Heparin-binding EGF-like growth factor protects intestinal stem cells from injury in a rat model of necrotizing enterocolitis. Lab Invest 2012;92(3):331–44.
45. Frost BL, Jilling T, Caplan MS. The importance of pro-inflammatory signaling in neonatal necrotizing enterocolitis. Semin Perinatol 2008;32(2):100–6.
46. Caplan MS, Simon D, Jilling T. The role of PAF, TLR, and the inflammatory response in neonatal necrotizing enterocolitis. Semin Pediatr Surg 2005;14(3): 145–51.
47. MacKendrick W, Caplan M. Necrotizing enterocolitis. New thoughts about pathogenesis and potential treatments. Pediatr Clin North Am 1993;40(5):1047–59.
48. Kliegman RM. The relationship of neonatal feeding practices and the pathogenesis and prevention of necrotizing enterocolitis. Pediatrics 2003;111(3):671–2.
49. Anderson DM, Kliegman RM. The relationship of neonatal alimentation practices to the occurrence of endemic necrotizing enterocolitis. Am J Perinatol 1991;8(1):62–7.
50. Kennedy KA, Tyson JE, Chamnanvanakij S. Rapid versus slow rate of advancement of feedings for promoting growth and preventing necrotizing enterocolitis in parenterally fed low-birth-weight infants. Cochrane Database Syst Rev 2000; 2:CD001241.
51. Morgan J, Young L, McGuire W. Delayed introduction of progressive enteral feeds to prevent necrotising enterocolitis in very low birth weight infants. Cochrane Database Syst Rev 2011;3:CD001970.

52. Morgan J, Young L, McGuire W. Slow advancement of enteral feed volumes to prevent necrotising enterocolitis in very low birth weight infants. Cochrane Database Syst Rev 2011;3:CD001241.
53. Rayyis SF, Ambalavanan N, Wright L, et al. Randomized trial of "slow" versus "fast" feed advancements on the incidence of necrotizing enterocolitis in very low birth weight infants. J Pediatr 1999;134(3):293–7.
54. Kamitsuka MD, Horton MK, Williams MA. The incidence of necrotizing enterocolitis after introducing standardized feeding schedules for infants between 1250 and 2500 grams and less than 35 weeks of gestation. Pediatrics 2000;105(2):379–84.
55. McCallie KR, Lee HC, Mayer O, et al. Improved outcomes with a standardized feeding protocol for very low birth weight infants. J Perinatol 2011;31(Suppl 1): S61–7.
56. McGuire W, Anthony MY. Donor human milk versus formula for preventing necrotising enterocolitis in preterm infants: systematic review. Arch Dis Child Fetal Neonatal Ed 2003;88(1):F11–4.
57. Boyd CA, Quigley MA, Brocklehurst P. Donor breast milk versus infant formula for preterm infants: systematic review and meta-analysis. Arch Dis Child Fetal Neonatal Ed 2007;92(3):F169–75.
58. Kuschel CA, Harding JE. Multicomponent fortified human milk for promoting growth in preterm infants. Cochrane Database Syst Rev 2004;1:CD000343.
59. Sullivan S, Schanler RJ, Kim JH, et al. An exclusively human milk-based diet is associated with a lower rate of necrotizing enterocolitis than a diet of human milk and bovine milk-based products. J Pediatr 2010;156(4):562–7, e1.
60. Singh R, Visintainer PF, Frantz ID 3rd, et al. Association of necrotizing enterocolitis with anemia and packed red blood cell transfusions in preterm infants. J Perinatol 2011;31(3):176–82.
61. Weintraub AS, Ferrara L, Deluca L, et al. Antenatal antibiotic exposure in preterm infants with necrotizing enterocolitis. J Perinatol 2011. [Epub ahead of print].
62. Kliegman RM. Neonatal necrotizing enterocolitis: bridging the basic science with the clinical disease. J Pediatr 1990;117(5):833–5.
63. Christensen RD, Wiedmeier SE, Baer VL, et al. Antecedents of Bell stage III necrotizing enterocolitis. J Perinatol 2010;30(1):54–7.
64. Kennedy J, Holt CL, Ricketts RR. The significance of portal vein gas in necrotizing enterocolitis. Am Surg 1987;53(4):231–4.
65. Young C, Sharma R, Handfield M, et al. Biomarkers for infants at risk for necrotizing enterocolitis: clues to prevention? Pediatr Res 2009;65(5 Pt 2):91R–7R.
66. Bell MJ, Ternberg JL, Feigin RD, et al. Neonatal necrotizing enterocolitis. Therapeutic decisions based upon clinical staging. Ann Surg 1978;187(1):1–7.
67. Ein SH, Marshall DG, Girvan D. Peritoneal drainage under local anesthesia for perforations from necrotizing enterocolitis. J Pediatr Surg 1977;12(6):963–7.
68. Moss RL, Dimmitt RA, Barnhart DC, et al. Laparotomy versus peritoneal drainage for necrotizing enterocolitis and perforation. N Engl J Med 2006;354(21):2225–34.
69. Rees CM, Eaton S, Kiely EM, et al. Peritoneal drainage or laparotomy for neonatal bowel perforation? A randomized controlled trial. Ann Surg 2008;248(1):44–51.
70. Stringer MD, Brereton RJ, Drake DP, et al. Recurrent necrotizing enterocolitis. J Pediatr Surg 1993;28(8):979–81.
71. O'Connor A, Sawin RS. High morbidity of enterostomy and its closure in premature infants with necrotizing enterocolitis. Arch Surg 1998;133(8):875–80.
72. Horwitz JR, Lally KP, Cheu HW, et al. Complications after surgical intervention for necrotizing enterocolitis: a multicenter review. J Pediatr Surg 1995;30(7):994–8 [discussion: 998–9].

73. Henry MC, Moss RL. Neonatal necrotizing enterocolitis. Semin Pediatr Surg 2008; 17(2):98–109.
74. Duro D, Kalish LA, Johnston P, et al. Risk factors for intestinal failure in infants with necrotizing enterocolitis: a Glaser Pediatric Research Network study. J Pediatr 2010;157(2):203–8, e1.
75. Andorsky DJ, Lund DP, Lillehei CW, et al. Nutritional and other postoperative management of neonates with short bowel syndrome correlates with clinical outcomes. J Pediatr 2001;139(1):27–33.
76. Arnold M, Moore SW, Sidler D, et al. Long-term outcome of surgically managed necrotizing enterocolitis in a developing country. Pediatr Surg Int 2010;26(4): 355–60.
77. Peyret B, Collardeau S, Touzet S, et al. Prevalence of liver complications in children receiving long-term parenteral nutrition. Eur J Clin Nutr 2011;65(6):743–9.
78. Duro D, Mitchell PD, Kalish LA, et al. Risk factors for parenteral nutrition-associated liver disease following surgical therapy for necrotizing enterocolitis: a Glaser Pediatric Research Network Study [corrected]. J Pediatr Gastroenterol Nutr 2011;52(5):595–600.
79. Hintz SR, Kendrick DE, Stoll BJ, et al. Neurodevelopmental and growth outcomes of extremely low birth weight infants after necrotizing enterocolitis. Pediatrics 2005;115(3):696–703.
80. Stevenson DK, Kerner JA, Malachowski N, et al. Late morbidity among survivors of necrotizing enterocolitis. Pediatrics 1980;66(6):925–7.
81. Mshvildadze M, Neu J. Probiotics and prevention of necrotizing enterocolitis. Early Hum Dev 2009;85(Suppl 10):S71–4.
82. Deshpande G, Rao S, Patole S. Probiotics for prevention of necrotising enterocolitis in preterm neonates with very low birthweight: a systematic review of randomised controlled trials. Lancet 2007;369(9573):1614–20.
83. Coursodon CF, Dvorak B. Epidermal growth factor and necrotizing enterocolitis. Curr Opin Pediatr 2012;24(2):160–4.
84. Feng J, Besner GE. Heparin-binding epidermal growth factor-like growth factor promotes enterocyte migration and proliferation in neonatal rats with necrotizing enterocolitis. J Pediatr Surg 2007;42(1):214–20.
85. Feng J, El-Assal ON, Besner GE. Heparin-binding epidermal growth factor-like growth factor reduces intestinal apoptosis in neonatal rats with necrotizing enterocolitis. J Pediatr Surg 2006;41(4):742–7 [discussion: 742–7].
86. Feng J, El-Assal ON, Besner GE. Heparin-binding epidermal growth factor-like growth factor decreases the incidence of necrotizing enterocolitis in neonatal rats. J Pediatr Surg 2006;41(1):144–9 [discussion: 144–9].
87. Radulescu A, Zhang HY, Yu X, et al. Heparin-binding epidermal growth factor-like growth factor overexpression in transgenic mice increases resistance to necrotizing enterocolitis. J Pediatr Surg 2010;45(10):1933–9.
88. Radulescu A, Yu X, Orvets ND, et al. Deletion of the heparin-binding epidermal growth factor-like growth factor gene increases susceptibility to necrotizing enterocolitis. J Pediatr Surg 2010;45(4):729–34.

Anorectal Malformations

Richard S. Herman, MD, Daniel H. Teitelbaum, MD*

KEYWORDS

- Anorectal malformation • Imperforate anus • Perineal fistula
- Neonatal bowel obstruction • VACTERL association • Congenital anomaly

KEY POINTS

- Workup of patients with anorectal malformations should begin with a thorough physical examination.
- Ruling out significant associated anomalies is necessary before initial surgical intervention.
- The type of lesions, high versus low, has a significant impact on continence and long-term outcomes.
- Associated gynecologic problems are not uncommon and may not be picked up until puberty or later.

HISTORY

The first description of humans born with anorectal malformations (ARM) was described by Aristotle in the early third century BCE, and the earliest reports of treatment for such defects began to appear in the second century CE by Soranus, who described cutting the thin perineal membrane and then dilating it. There was little progress in the treatment or description of ARM until the late seventeenth century, when Saviard attempted to treat a high lesion by plunging a trocar through the perineum. About a century later the first dissection to a blind-ending colon was described by Bell, who also described the associated anatomic defects of rectovesical and rectovaginal fistulas.[1] However, it is likely that during this time most of these infants died, and surgeons were unable to achieve successful treatment. In the late 1700s inguinal colostomies were first reported; however, most of these procedures resulted in death and this procedure was thus used only as a final option.[2] In 1835 Amussat[3] performed the first proctoplasty, but destroyed most of the sphincter complex during the procedure. From the mid-1900s to the early 1980s passage of the rectum through a puborectalis ring was used, as described by Stephens.[4] A potential disadvantage of this

The authors have nothing to disclose.

Section of Pediatric Surgery, University of Michigan, Ann Arbor, MI, USA

* Division of Pediatric Surgery, C.S. Mott Children's Hospital, 1540 East Hospital Drive, SPC 4211, Ann Arbor, MI 48109-4211.

E-mail address: dttlbm@med.umich.edu

Clin Perinatol 39 (2012) 403–422

doi:10.1016/j.clp.2012.04.001

0095-5108/12/$ – see front matter © 2012 Elsevier Inc. All rights reserved.

perinatology.theclinics.com

approach was that it involved a blind dissection around the urethra and prostate gland. The posterior sagittal anorectoplasty was described by DeVries and Peña[5] in 1982, and is still used today. In 2000 Georgeson and colleagues[6] described the laparoscopic approach to imperforate anus.

EPIDEMIOLOGY

Anorectal malformations are one of the causes of bowel obstruction in the neonate. However, the incidence is rare, occurring in about 1 in every 4000 to 5000 live births, with about one-third being isolated and the remainder associated with other congenital abnormalities.[7] There is a slight male predominance and certain familial associations have been described[8,9]; however, there has been no discernible identifier regarding a possible cause. In addition, ARM have been associated with various genetic conditions (see later discussion). The most common lesion seen in males is a rectourethral fistula, with the most common in females being a rectovestibular fistula.

EMBRYOLOGY

Anorectal malformations occur secondary to abnormalities in the development of the hindgut, which gives rise to the descending colon, rectum, and the upper part of the anal canal, the lining of bladder, and the urethra. The hindgut will enter into the posterior region of the cloaca. The fetal cloaca is an endoderm-lined cavity covered at its ventral portion by ectoderm. The junction of the endoderm and ectoderm is termed the cloacal membrane. During development the urorectal septum will divide the area between the hindgut and the allantois, ultimately forming the perineal body. The allantois is an endodermal outpouching of the yolk sac, with its specialized mesenchyme that lies close to the cloaca and becomes the umbilical cord. During the seventh week of development the cloacal membrane separates, creating the anal opening for the hindgut and ventral opening for the urogenital sinus, with the perineal body forming between the two. The posterior aspect closes with ectoderm and then is recanalized 2 weeks later. An evolving theory on the etiology of these defects has occurred, with current thinking being that the development of imperforate anus is caused by lack of recanalization during the ninth week of gestation and ectopic positioning of the anal opening in the cloaca. The extent of anorectal defects relates to the degree of development in the posterior aspect of the cloaca. Smaller defects will lead to distal presentations such as covered anus and anocutaneous fistula, whereas larger defects will lead to more proximal anomalies such as urogenital fistula or cloacal malformations.[10,11]

GENETICS

In addition to the multitude of genetic syndromes that have been associated with ARM, recent investigations have evaluated possible genetic causes of ARM. Overall, the incidence of anorectal malformations in the setting of a genetic disease is about 5% to 10%. Trisomy 21 and a microdeletion of the chromosome 22q11.2 are the 2 most frequent. However, anorectal malformations have been reported in association with mutations in almost all chromosomes.[12] Towne-Brock syndrome, FG syndrome (Opitz-Kaveggia syndrome), Johanson-Blizzard syndrome, Kaufman-McKusick syndrome, Trisomies 8 and 21, and Fragile X syndrome are some of the genetic syndromes that have been shown to have associated ARM.[11] Trisomy 21 differs from most of the other genetic diseases in that the associated ARM is usually without an associated fistula. In addition to genetic disorders, recent literature has begun to identify a familial inheritance pattern for ARM. For those patients with a rectovestibular or rectoperineal fistula, almost 15% had a positive family history for an ARM.[13] Thus, families of a child with an ARM should be advised that compared with the regular population, their subsequent children or the patient's offspring are at increased risk for an ARM.

Recent animal studies have begun to investigate specific genetic defects associated with ARMs. Three candidate genes are the sonic hedgehog, Wnt5a, and Skt. Suda and colleagues[14] demonstrated that an Sd mouse strain with a short tail and a mutation in chromosome 2 contains an Skt^{GT} mutation with a 100% incidence of ARM. The investigators' focus was to analyze the cloacal plate of this mutated mouse embryo. In their model they noticed that the cloacal plate failed to elongate secondary to a defect in the dorsal region, leading to a thickening of the surrounding tissues. The resultant mutation consisted of a phenotype whereby these mice developed a fistula between the rectum and urogenital tract; however, the mechanism by which the Skt gene affects ARM is still under investigation.

Sonic Hedgehog Homolog (SHH) signaling is a main pathway for gut development in all animals. Mice with mutations in SHH develop a phenotype consistent with an ARM. Zhang and colleagues[15] investigated ARM mutations in human SHH signaling by processing tissues samples taken from patients with a variety of ARM anomalies during surgical repair. Their study showed a decreased level of SHH in patients with a high ARM, but no significant differences comparing low ARM and controls. Another protein, GLI-2, which is involved in SHH signaling, was lower in the patients with low lesions compared with the control group. That there was a difference in the concentration of SHH in the high and low ARM groups, suggesting that the pathogenesis differed among high and low lesions.

Another model for creating anorectal malformations in mice was based on inactivation of fibroblast growth factor 10. It was postulated that this is an effector downstream from the Wnt5a gene. During the investigation of Wnt5a, investigators identified fistula formation during early development, suggesting that it is not the obstruction that causes fistula formation but rather the gene mutation.[16] It is clear that the pathogenesis of ARM has many influencing factors and now that animal models are available, the pathogenesis and ultimate prevention of this disorder may be identified.

DIAGNOSIS AND WORKUP

Prenatal diagnosis has both low specificity and low sensitivity. Occasionally a dilated colon can be seen but is not specific for ARM. Other signs that may indicate ARM are oligohydramnios and a distended vagina. It is more likely that associated anomalies will be picked up prenatally.[17]

After birth, most ARMs should be identified on the initial newborn examination. After the diagnosis of an ARM is made, as with any congenital anomaly the next step is to perform a thorough physical examination, which should focus on not only the presence of an anal, vaginal, and urethral opening but also their relative position on the perineum.

Once the diagnosis of an imperforate anus is made, assessment for the presence of a fistula should be performed. The fistula can reside from just anterior to the normal position of the anus to anywhere along the median raphe extending to the corona of the penile shaft. A careful examination of the urethral meatus, checking for meconium staining, is important and would indicate a fistula to the urogenital system. It is possible that it may take up to 24 hours for signs of a fistula to become evident. Therefore, the absence of these findings during the first day of life does not eliminate the possibility of a coexistent fistula. A bucket-handle type anomaly (**Fig. 1**) suggests an intermediate to low depth of the ARM. Squamous epithelium or meconium on microscopic examination of the urine is another sign indicating a fistula to the urinary system.

To understand the anomaly present in a female, one must first understand the normal position of each of the involved structures. The anal opening should be one-third of the distance between the coccyx and the fourchette. In addition, the tuberosities of the pelvis should be aligned with the normal anal opening. Parasagittal muscle fibers are located on either side of the midline and form the buttock groove. A paucity of these muscle fibers is an indication of a higher lesion. In the absence of an anal opening, one should search for a fistula more proximally, in the perineum up to and including within the fourchette. The actual number of orifices is another important diagnosis to pick up on physical examination, and can often be quite difficult in the neonate. The insertion of probes into the different orifices will often help to make the diagnosis and can help differentiate between the different types of anomalies. This action requires the physician to spread the introitus open, and inspect for individual urethral, vaginal, and potentially rectal fistula openings. Classically a fistula will track posteriorly when probed. The finding of a single opening on the perineum is consistent with a cloacal anomaly (see later discussion).

After a thorough physical examination, radiologic studies can help to determine a high from a low lesion and assist with surgical planning. The inversion radiograph, described by Wangensteen and Rice,[18] shows the distance between the distal gas bubbles in the colon and the perineal opening. Later, Narasimharao and colleagues[19] refined this technique by using a prone cross-table lateral radiograph (**Fig. 2**). In this series, the patients were placed in the prone position for a minimum of 3 minutes. These studies should be performed at 24 hours after birth to allow enteric gas to reach the most distal area of the colon; otherwise a high lesion might be suggested because the colonic gas has not yet had time to reach the distal pouch. One should avoid a delay of workup beyond 24 hours, as this has led to perforation of the proximal colon in some neonates. If the modified invertogram shows air extending below the level of the coccyx, a lower anomaly is suggested. In this latter case, and without other major

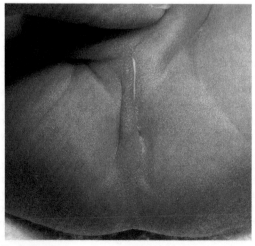

Fig. 1. Bucket-handle deformity.

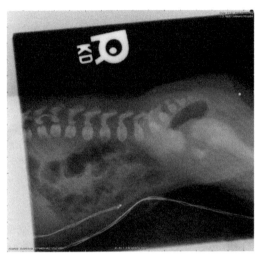

Fig. 2. A cross-table lateral radiograph.

anomalies, one might approach this anomaly by performing a primary posterior sagittal anorectoplasty without a protective colostomy, based on the surgeon's experience.

After initial evaluation and radiologic imaging, one must next look for other congenital anomalies, especially those that could be life threatening. About 50% to 67% of all anorectal malformations are associated with other anomalies,[20] including vertebral anomalies, cardiac lesions, trachea and esophageal abnormalities, and renal and limb defects (known collectively by the acronym VACTERL).

Cardiac

The reported incidence of patients with ARM and cardiac anomalies ranges from 10% to as high as 30%; however, most anomalies will not require urgent treatment.[21] Initial management should include an echocardiogram, and these results should determine the next steps in treatment. Atrial septal defects and ventricular septal defects have been the most common findings.[22]

Spinal and Vertebral

Spinal and vertebral anomalies are the most prevalent associations with ARM, with an overall incidence ranging between one-third and one-half of all ARM patients. Tethered cord is the most common spinal abnormality and occurs in about 20% to 30% of patients.[23,24] Once a tethered cord is identified, the patient should be evaluated by a pediatric neurosurgeon, as many of the patients may require surgical intervention. Diagnosis of these anomalies is usually via spinal ultrasonography in young infants; however, once the child is past the age of 1 year, magnetic resonance imaging (MRI) is often needed. MRI is now considered a valuable tool in evaluating associated spinal and sacral anomalies in patients with ARM. However, a screening ultrasonogram does not require a general anesthetic, and it is preferred that MRI be withheld for those infants with abnormal sonographic findings.[25] Different types of vertebral anomalies include hemivertebrae, scoliosis, butterfly vertebrae, hemisacrum, and diastematomyelia, with the most common being spina bifida and fusion defects of the lumbosacral region.[26]

The sacral ratio described by Levitt and Peña[2] is a good predictor of continence. Patients with ratios less than 0.3 are usually incontinent whereas those who have ratios closer to 1.0 are usually continent (**Fig. 3**).[2,27] Currarino's triad, which includes a presacral mass, anorectal malformation, and sacral defects, has a strong familial inheritance pattern, and should be considered in patients with ARM.[28]

Finally, the degree of the abnormalities of the sacrum has been shown to a have a strong correlation with postoperative function and complications. For those patients who have more than 4 intact sacral elements, postoperative assessments demonstrate satisfying results.[29] Patients with more than 2 missing sacral vertebrae, hemisacral defects, or tethered cord had significantly worse bowel function scores.[30] In addition, Peña[31] showed that those with an absent sacrum were observed to have urinary incontinence.

Tracheoesophageal Fistula

Esophageal atresia (EA) and tracheoesophageal fistula (TEF) occur in about 5% to 10% of patients with ARM.[26] The diagnosis of an esophageal atresia can be suggested with a routine chest radiograph during the attempted passage of a nasogastric tube. The timing and the order for operative repair of a TEF/EA with an ARM depends

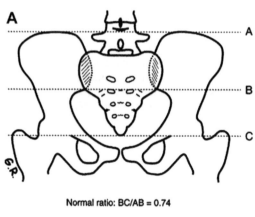

Normal ratio: BC/AB = 0.74

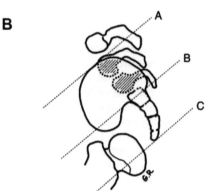

Normal ratio: BC/AB = 0.77

Fig. 3. Anterior-posterior (*A*) and lateral (*B*) sacral ratios. (*Courtesy of* Peña A, Levitt MA, Cincinnati Children's Hospital.)

greatly on what procedure needs to be done, cardiac status, potential need for a colostomy for the ARM, and the timing of such procedures with the TEF. Often these procedures can be done in close proximity to each other, or concurrently. Typically the more life threatening lesion, the TEF, should be approached first.

Genitourinary Associations

The reported incidence of genitourinary anomalies in patients with ARM ranges from 33% to almost 50%. This incidence does not include fistulas to the urinary system (see later discussion). The most common anomaly overall is reflux, and the most common high lesion is renal agenesis. Other anomalies included horseshoe kidney, multicystic kidney, ectopic kidney, hypoplasia/dysplasia, and obstruction. Chronic renal failure is estimated to occur in 2% to 6% of ARM patients, and has been a cause of significant morbidity and mortality.[26,32]

Urinary continence is often not considered as a potential problem in patients with ARM, but should be considered in any child after a pull-through who has fecal incontinence. For patients who have complex anomalies, 39% will have a lumbosacral or spinal cord anomaly and of these, 43% will suffer from lower urinary tract dysfunction.[33] The actual mechanism for bladder/urinary dysfunction is poorly understood but is thought to arise from a neuropathic origin. Urinary incontinence leads to significant morbidity in these patients. It is postulated that frequent urinary tract infections, often a consequence of reflux or other renal anomalies, can be a cause of incontinence. In addition, nerve injury during reconstruction or due to sacral agenesis may lead to incontinence. In a study by Boemers and colleagues,[34] urinary incontinence was seen in 18% of patients. Senel and colleagues[35] recently reported a 25% incidence of severe uropathology in ARM patients. The earlier bladder dysfunction is detected, the better is the chance of preventing progression to complete incontinence.

Because of the high incidence of associated renal problems with ARM, all patients should undergo a screening renal ultrasonogram. A voiding cystourethrogram should be performed in those with upper renal tract anomalies, lumbosacral and spinal abnormalities, or frequent urinary tract infections. Urodynamics should be assessed in all patients with complex high ARM. Those who have documented issues will need long-term follow-up, as untreated urologic problems can lead to renal failure and mortality.[35]

Gynecologic Associations

Although gynecologic problems are common in ARM, most of them may not be diagnosed until puberty or adulthood. Early diagnosis is important to plan for optimal treatment through puberty and into adulthood. In a review by Levitt and colleagues,[36] 17% of patients with a rectovestibular fistula, the most common anorectal malformation seen in females, had an associated gynecologic anomaly. Anomalies included multiple or absent vagina, cervix, and uterus. Vaginal atresia is a rare type of gynecologic anomaly, seen in 7% of patients with a rectovestibular fistula,[36] which can easily be missed and confused with either an imperforate anus without a fistula or a rectovestibular fistula with normal urethral and vaginal openings. One syndrome in which vaginal atresia is a key component is the Mayer-Rokitansky syndrome, whereby 75% of patients have a vaginal atresia and the remaining 25% a short vaginal pouch. These patients always have a 46XX genotype and make up 15% of females with primary amenorrhea.[37] Such patients usually have a good prognosis if diagnosed appropriately.[38] The diagnosis of congenital gynecologic anomalies in the past has been accomplished using a combination of physical examination (with or without anesthesia), ultrasonography, hysterosalpingography, and laparoscopy. Reports have shown that MRI is a valuable adjunct in diagnosing and differentiating upper gyneco-logic anomalies before surgical intervention.[39] Evaluation for hydrocolpos, seen with cloacal defects, needs to be done early in the neonatal period (or even prenatally) and again at the time of definitive repair when a complete evaluation of the anatomy can be performed. Because issues may arise later during puberty or at the time of planned delivery, long-term follow-up is mandatory.

The next sections describe the specific anomalies present and their various treat-ment options. The anomalies are divided by gender, starting with lesions in the male. In either case, the initial step for all patients with possible defects is a thorough perineal examination.

LESIONS IN THE MALE

Workup for males with ARM (**Fig. 4**) begins by classifying patients into low-lying lesions or higher lesions, as these have important clinical implications with regard to their treatment and prognosis for long-term outcomes, especially with respect to continence. The best chance for continence is found in those children with low lesions, such as rectoperineal fistulas. Those with intermediate lesions, such as the rectoure-thral fistula with insertion on the bulbar aspect of the urethra, have moderate chances for continence. Those with relatively high lesions, such as a rectourethral fistula to the prostatic urethra or bladder itself, have very little chance for fecal continence.

Imperforate Anus Without Fistula

In this lesion the perineum is completely covered with no identifiable opening. Poten-tially, this develops either because of hypertrophy of the genital folds or because of failure of perforation of the anal membrane, the more rare occurrence.[40] The anus is

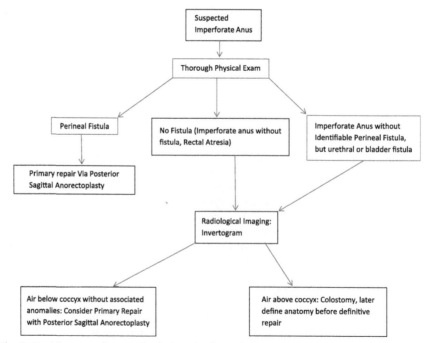

Fig. 4. Decision-tree diagram for lesions in the male.

located in the normal anatomic location, with good preservation of muscles and sacrum. The urethra and rectum share a thin common wall, and about one-half of these patients will have Trisomy 21. Diagnosis is made by the absence of a fistula and gas noted at a low or intermediate position on radiologic image. In the case of infants with Trisomy 21, a biopsy of the distal portion of the rectum needs to be performed to rule out aganglionosis.

Treatment

After ruling out other associated diseases, the initial decision in the treatment of any ARM is whether to perform a colostomy or to proceed with primary repair (see **Fig. 4**). This decision should be made in conjunction with a post–24-hour prone lateral radiograph to help delineate the termination of the rectum. For patients with an imperforate anus and no fistula, the level of air seen on the prone lateral radiograph may offer useful information. If air is visualized below the coccyx, a primary repair via a posterior sagittal anorectoplasty (PSARP) can be achieved. If air terminates above the level of the coccyx, a diversion colostomy should be performed. A definitive determination of the distal extent cannot always be obtained. In such situations, the threshold to perform a colostomy should be quite low, as this is the safest approach.

If a colostomy has been created, a colostogram should be performed before definitive repair to better delineate the anatomy. The colostogram injection should be performed through a Foley catheter in the colostomy while placing gentle traction on the inflated Foley balloon. This approach, as advanced by the Cincinnati group, will increase diagnostic and anatomic accuracy.[41] Uncertainty of the anatomy increases the risk of injury to important structures such as the ureter, bladder, urethra, and vas deferens.[42] Because most of these lesions are low, most should be able to be completed with a PSARP; however, in the case of lesions that terminate higher in the pelvis an abdominal approach should be used, typically via laparoscopy.

Rectoperineal Fistula

Rectoperineal fistula is also referred to as a covered anus, anal membrane, or anteriorly mislocated anus.[43] In this lesion the majority of the rectum is located normally within the muscular complexes, but the most distal aspect of the rectum lies anteriorly. The fistulous opening can be located anywhere from just anterior to the normal position of the rectum along the midline up to the shaft of the penis, including the median raphe of the scrotum. Perineal inspection is the only diagnostic modality that is necessary in these patients. These fistulas are often stenotic. Specks of meconium can help to localize the fistulous opening (**Fig. 5**).

Treatment

When a fistula to the perineum is present, a colostomy is rarely required because definitive repair can be performed in the newborn period, using either the lithotomy or the prone position. Care must be taken during the dissection as the anterior surface of the rectum and the urethra share a common wall, without a plane of dissection. A Foley catheter in place during the procedure can help identify the urethra, and should always be used.

Rectourethral Fistula (to the Bulbar Urethra)

In this lesion the rectum terminates above the bulbospongiosus muscle. The fistula can either be a narrow connection to the urethra, or slightly higher up with a wider fistula. Superficial to the rectum exists a voluntary muscle complex, which with perineal nerve stimulation shows good contraction. A normal internal anal sphincter does not exist in these patients, but a normal sacrum and anal dimple are usually

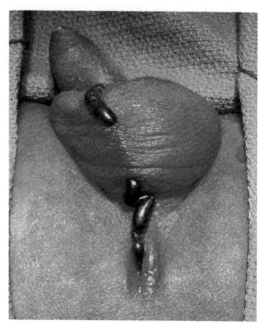

Fig. 5. Meconium tracking along the fistula in a low imperforate anus in the male.

present.[43] The rectum and urethra share a common wall that is longer the lower the fistula. Because of the risk of urine backwashing into the rectum, one should monitor electrolytes in infants with a rectourethral fistula. If the bicarbonate level declines to below 20 mEq/L, infants should receive oral sodium bicarbonate to compensate. This level will abate once the fistula is ligated.

Treatment

In general, a diverting colostomy is performed. As already mentioned, a colostogram should be obtained and is helpful in planning definitive operative repair. The incision is again via a posterior sagittal approach. In the case of a rectobulbar fistula the rectum being found just below the levators, the risk of urinary injury is lower than in the setting of a higher lesion. It is noteworthy that during repair the urethra and rectum share a common wall, which must be approached via an anterior submucosal dissection on the rectum. After separation, the fistula is closed with interrupted monofilament sutures. The rectum is then circumferentially dissected free of adjacent blood supply until adequate length is achieved. The levator complex is then reapproximated posteriorly and superficially over the rectum. The rectum is anastomosed in the center of the muscle complex and the perineum is closed. The dissection and reconstruction are guided using a muscle stimulator, being careful to bring the rectum through the external sphincter muscle complex.

Rectal Atresia

Rectal atresia is an uncommon malformation whereby the rectum is in the normal anatomic position. The sacrum and muscle complexes are normal, and an anus is present in the normal location. The rectum can terminate at any level, but a fibrous cord usually connects to the sacrum or distal bowel. The upper portion is dilated. The anal canal is normal for about 1 to 2 cm. Diagnosis is made with digital rectal examination whereby one encounters an obstruction.

Treatment
The treatment of rectal atresia is performed via a posterior approach and entails identifying the proximal rectal pouch, opening it up, and performing an end-to-end anastomosis to the distal anal canal. The proximal portion is usually dilated whereas the distal portion is often small and narrow. There is variability as to whether the atresia consists of a short membrane or a dense fibrous band. It is important to identify a potential presacral mass during this procedure (ie, Currarino's triad, though much more common with an anteriorly displaced anal opening) and, if present, remove it during the operation. Because these patients typically have normal muscle and nerve function, meticulous repair of the sphincter complex is essential.[43]

High Lesions

High rectourethral fistula
In this defect the fistula opens onto the urethra posteriorly. There is no internal anal sphincter, and the muscle quality of the external sphincter is poor. As a result, incontinence is present in the majority of patients. In addition, there is often an abnormally developed sacrum. On physical examination, classically there is no identifiable rectum, a flat perineum, a poorly formed midline groove, and a barely visible dimple. Radiologic examination may demonstrate air in the bladder. The final diagnosis and level of the fistula can be made with a colostogram. Because of the high association of urinary anomalies, a retrograde urethrogram and possibly cystoscopy may be performed, which will corroborate the findings of the colostogram.[43]

Treatment The repair of this defect is similar to that for rectobulbar fistula. A diverting colostomy should be done and a colostogram performed before repair. The approach is again via a posterior sagittal incision. The rectum found near the level of the coccyx and the fistula tract will insert into the urethra near the prostate. This operation is considerably more complicated than in the setting of a rectobulbar fistula, and the risk of injury to the genitourinary tract can be higher. Traction sutures are an integral part of performing a safe procedure. Multiple fibrous bands and vessels attach to the rectum in the pelvis, and must be divided or else one may not have sufficient length to bring the rectum through without tension to the perineum (**Fig. 6**). At times, further mobilization must be done via an abdominal approach. As with rectobulbar fistula, dissecting in the submucosal plane of the rectum will help to separate the common wall between the prostatic urethra and rectum. Approximation and repair is the same as for rectobulbar fistula. A Foley should be left in place for 5 days after the procedure. Feeds can begin on the first postoperative day, as patients generally have a diverting colostomy.

Laparoscopic repairs
An alternative approach that works quite well for patients with high lesions is a laparoscopic approach. In this case, the infant is placed at the end of the operating table (**Fig. 7**). Three laparoscopic ports are placed, although a fourth may be necessary. To gain better exposure to the distal rectum, a transcutaneous stay stitch is placed around the bladder to suspend it anteriorly. The peritoneum around the rectum is opened, being careful to avoid the vas deferens, ureters, and bladder. The dissection can be lengthy, but continues distally until the fistula is identified (**Fig. 8**). The fistula can be ligated with sutures or an endoloop. The rectum is then mobilized until sufficient length is attained. At this point, one surgeon moves to the perineum while the assistant holds up the legs in a lithotomy position. A limited (approximately the size of the eventual rectum) vertical incision is made, guided by a muscle stimulator, so that it is centered where the neorectum will be placed. Once the dissection is carried

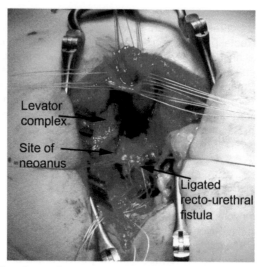

Fig. 6. Intraoperative photo of a posterior sagittal rectoanoplasty.

through the vertical muscle complex, a Veress needle is placed with an STEP trocar sheath (Covidien Corp., Mansfield, MA, USA). Visualization internally is used to make sure that the trocar goes through the midportion of the levators and posterior to the urethra. The sheath is dilated by placement of a 12-mm port size, the rectum is brought through the levator complex, and an anastomosis is performed.

A critical question is whether the laparoscopic approach affords similar results to a PSARP in both function and outcome. Since the first report by Georgeson and colleagues[6] in 2000, many other studies have examined the potential advantages of the laparoscopic approach. Short-term data have shown that the laparoscopic approach appears to be at least equivalent to the standard open approach for ARM. However, long-term functional outcomes have yet to be determined[44] Moreover, because most of the lesions approached laparoscopically have high proximal fistulous connections, it is likely that the functional outcomes will be poor regardless

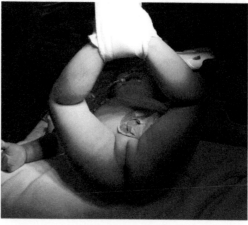

Fig. 7. Positioning of the patient for operative repair.

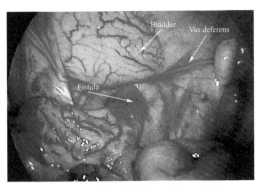

Fig. 8. Laparoscopic view showing bladder, fistula, and vas deferens.

of the approach. Bailez and colleagues[45,46] discussed the use of the laparoscopic approach for repair of rectovaginal fistulas in females and in males with high anorectal malformations, and concluded that the approach was effective. Although the laparoscopic procedure is a technically very viable approach, future studies on long-term outcomes and function are required.

Rectovesical fistula
With this lesion the fistulous tract enters the bladder. Many of the physical findings are similar to those seen for rectourethral fistula. Incontinence is likely secondary to poor development of levator muscle and external sphincter complex.

Treatment These patients are best approached via an abdominal approach, ideally laparoscopic (see earlier discussion). The fistula should be divided via the abdominal approach. Because this lesion is much higher there is a very short common wall, which makes division easier.

LESIONS IN THE FEMALE
Low Lesions

Imperforate anus without fistula, rectal atresia, and rectoperineal fistula
Essentially the diagnosis and treatment is similar to that described for the male patient. For the rectoperineal fistula, the majority of the rectum is in the normal position, with the lower part displaced anteriorly. These patients have a good prognosis for fecal continence. Two key aspects of the rectoperineal fistula are the length of the perineal body and the location of the anal opening in relation to the muscle complex. **Fig. 9** shows a suggested workup of female patients with these anomalies.

Rectovestibular Fistula

Rectovestibular fistula is the most common defect seen in female patients. Here, the rectum will usually terminate above the pubococcygeal line. A fine fistula with a length of 1 to 2 cm will enter the posterior aspect of the vestibule. A key important aspect of the examination is to ensure that there are 3 distinct openings: the urethra, the vagina, and the rectal fistula (**Fig. 10**). With this anomaly the fistula course is adjacent to the posterior wall of the vagina. A small percentage of patients with this defect will have 2 hemivaginas with a septum. The diagnosis of this defect is made by a thorough physical examination. Often the opening of the fistula can be difficult to find in the posterior aspect of the vestibule, and requires probing the distinct orifices to facilitate

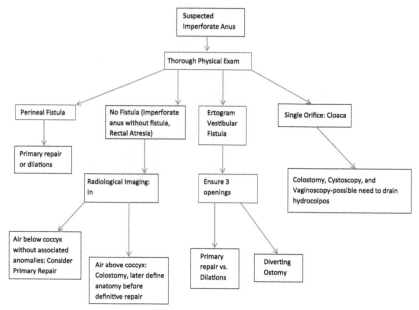

Fig. 9. Decision-tree diagram for lesions in the female.

identification. If the anatomy is not clear, a fistulogram may help define the anatomy as well as the length of the fistula and the level of the rectum. Vaginoscopy should be considered if the anatomy is unclear. Most these patients will have a good functional outcome.

Treatment

This defect is typically repaired without a diverting colostomy. If the fistula can be dilated and if the patient stools without evidence of obstruction, the child can be sent home with dilations, returning for definitive repair when older than 3 months.

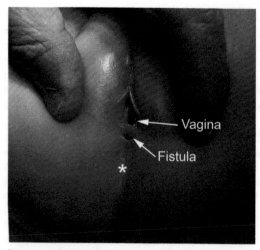

Fig. 10. Picture of a low imperforate anus in the female, showing 3 distinct orifices. * Represents site of normal anal opening.

Stooling is facilitated typically by the caregiver or parent performing twice-daily dilations with Hegar dilators that do not exceed #8 or #9 in size. For infants who are nursed, this should suffice. For infants receiving formula, the addition of polyethylene glycol (3500 molecular weight) should be added at a dose of 1 teaspoon in a bottle of formula each day. It is important to ensure that the rectum is truly emptying and that there is not a small amount of liquid stool passing around a distal obstruction.

The approach for this repair is also via a posterior sagittal approach. The incision must extend into the vestibule and around the fistula. Here the rectum and the posterior aspect of the vagina share a long common wall, which must be carefully separated (**Fig. 11**). Care is taken to avoid entry into the vagina or rectum, which could result in dehiscence, stricture, or development of a rectovaginal fistula.[47] Furthermore, one must be careful to fully dissect the rectum off the vaginal wall or there could be kinking of the rectum as the neoanus is formed. Once the dissection is complete, the rectum is sutured to its optimal position in the muscle complex and the perineum is then closed in multiple layers. Another approach is that advocated by Potts (**Fig. 12C**).[48] With this approach, a circumferential dissection is carried just around the fistula and distal rectum, separating it from the vaginal wall. A counterincision is made where the neoanus should be. Then, preserving the perineum, a forceps reaches through the neoanal incision above the muscle complex and grabs the dissected rectum, pulling it through posteriorly. Should there be a didelphys vagina, unification of the 2 hemivaginas can typically be performed with simple division of the membrane at the time of anoplasty.

Cloaca

Cloaca is the most complicated ARM, with one similar feature: the rectal fistula, vagina, and urethra all join into one cloaca, presenting as a single orifice on the perineum. In one defect the 3 structures insert in proper orientation into the cloaca, with the rectal fistula most posterior and the urethra most anterior. In this case it is still possible to have a shortened vagina, which may be either single or septated. In the second type of cloaca, the rectal fistula inserts between the 2 hemivaginas, entering more anteriorly onto the cloaca. These defects can also have an associated bifid uterus (uterus didelphys). The length of the common channel has significant prognosis for rectal continence and technical difficulty of the surgical repair. Patients having a common channel shorter than 3 cm have a good prognosis, whereas those with

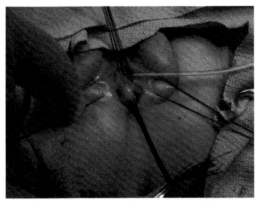

Fig. 11. Intraoperative dissection separating the common wall.

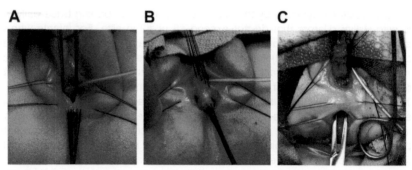

Fig. 12. Pott's approach to a posterior sagittal anoplasty. (*A*) Initial traction sutures during PSARP. (*B*) Dissection of common wall between vagina and rectum. (*C*) Intraoperative staged photo of a Potts repair.

a common channel longer than 3 cm have a more complicated defect and a far worse prognosis.[2] The immediate anatomic issues are not isolated to the cloaca. Frequently hydrocolpos exists, with fluid and secretions building up in the vaginal lumen, resulting in excessive distension that can lead to compression of the bladder trigone. This process causes a megacystis or even hydronephrosis, which at times may require emergent drainage of the vagina in the newborn period. The diagnosis of a cloaca is made on physical examination via identification of a single orifice, and further confirmation is made with ultrasonography. Determination of the size and location of the fistula can be done with a colostogram (after its creation) as well as with cystoscopy and vaginoscopy. A genitogram performed with contrast injection into the cloaca may also help to delineate the anatomy.

Treatment

As this is the most complicated of all ARM, its repair is often the most challenging. As with any of these malformations, a thorough understanding of the anatomy is vital before undertaking any surgical repair. Because the length of the common channel is a major influence on the ultimate repair, endoscopic evaluation of the common channel is the first step. All surgical cases should begin with an endoscopic examination, typically with a rigid cystoscope. The authors have found that placement of Fogarty catheters into each cavity (and properly labeling them) facilitates the surgery.

Cloacas with a short common channel (<3 cm) Defects with a common channel shorter than 3 cm can usually be repaired with the avoidance of an abdominal incision. A posterior sagittal incision is made and dissection is performed, usually encountering the rectum as the first structure. Complete exposure of the common channel is then performed, and one should confirm the length estimates already assessed during endoscopy. After the common channel is completely freed, the rectum is separated from the vagina. The entire urogenital tract is then mobilized and brought down as a single unit. Urogenital mobilization allows both structures to be brought down to the perineum as a single unit, decreasing morbidity such as development of a urethro-vaginal fistula.[49] Once completed, the urethral meatus and the vaginal introitus are anastomosed to the perineum. The rectum is anastomosed to the perineum, again in the center of the muscle complex. Finally, the former common channel is divided and used to create the labia. The remainder of the incision is then closed.

Cloacas with a long common channel (>3 cm) This defect typically requires a combined perineal and abdominal approach. The rectum and common channel are first identified, mobilized, and separated via a posterior sagittal approach. The abdominal approach will then be needed to complete the dissection and free the ureters, uterus, bladder, and vagina. The ureters should be protected with catheters as they run through the defect, and often need to be reimplanted into the bladder. Mobilization of the vagina to the perineum may require augmentation of the remnant vagina with colon interposition. The fallopian tubes need to be assessed for patency. If they are atretic they should be left alone, monitored, and reevaluated during puberty; if they are patent they can be anastomosed to the neovagina. If there are 2 hemivaginas present, both must be separated from the urinary tract and unified. If a vesicostomy is created, final repair is usually delayed until the patient is around 3 to 4 years of age.[2]

COMPLICATIONS AND LONG-TERM PROBLEMS

When discussing the complications and outcomes associated with ARMs, both short-term and long-term issues and function must be assessed. Some of the complications related directly to the surgical procedure are wound infections, which are usually limited and resolve with healing by secondary intention. Anal strictures, rectal prolapse (4%),[50] femoral nerve injury, and neurogenic bladder are other complications commonly encountered. For cloacal repairs, urethrovaginal fistulas, vaginal strictures, or fibrosis may be seen. In males, urologic injuries may be associated with dissection of a rectourethral fistula. In addition, megarectum, which can lead to motility and functional issues, can occur if a distal ostomy is not irrigated/evacuated well while awaiting surgical repair. When patients reach adulthood, problems with sexual dysfunction and constipation are observed.

The functional outcomes of ARM are often dependent on the type of lesion, with lower lesions having a better functional outcome than higher lesions. Those with lower lesions are, however, more likely to have issues with constipation, whereas those with higher lesions are more likely to have issues with fecal incontinence.[43] Issues with continence are often related to sensation, voluntary muscle control, or bowel motility. Almost all patients with ARM will have an altered sensation when it comes to stooling. Often their sensation is secondary to rectal distension because of the presence of stool. However, it is often possible that liquid stool will not be sensed, which will lead to soiling. Voluntary muscle control is also problematic, because this function usually relies on an element of sensation that is not available to patients following ARM repair. Reports of continence have ranged as high as 90% in patients with low malformations to as low as 10% in patients with long-segment cloacas and bladder neck fistulas.[2,51]

Most reports relate to the short term and there is little follow-up into adulthood. For patients suffering from fecal incontinence, a bowel regimen program will often help control soiling episodes. Patients benefit most from a comprehensive program, with nursing, surgeons, and behavioral pediatricians working together. If long-term incontinence is identified, the child will benefit most from the placement of an appendicostomy for daily colonic washouts. Use of such a program can dramatically improve outcomes.[52]

Finally, constipation remains a significant problem in patients following repair of ARM. If untreated, constipation can lead to overflow pseudoincontinence and poor bowel motility secondary to megacolon. Most patients with constipation following treatment of an ARM should be managed medically with stool softeners or enemas. Occasionally a child may require an appendicostomy. When evaluating a patient for constipation, one must ensure that a stricture has not formed.[53] One encouraging aspect is that observed by Rintala and Lindahl,[54] who showed that constipation will usually dissipate when a child reaches puberty, although the mechanisms of this phenomenon are unclear at present.

SUMMARY

Anorectal malformations exist in a wide range of complexity, and can often present as part of a genetic syndrome. These defects may be isolated or may present with other associated congenital anomalies. The success of their treatment is determined by the type of defect, the neuromuscular deficits associated with the ARM, the surgical procedure and techniques used, and aggressive postoperative follow-up and management.

REFERENCES

1. Holschneider AM, Hutson JM, editors. Anorectal malformations in children. Berlin: Springer; 2006. p. 3.
2. Peña A, Levitt M. Anorectal malformations. Pediatric surgery. 6th edition; 2006. p. 1566. Chapter 101.
3. Amussat. Histoire d'une operation d'anus practique avec success par un nouveau procede. Paris 1853.
4. Stephens FD. Malformations of the anus. Aust N Z J Surg 1953;23(1):9–24.
5. deVries PA, Peña A. Posterior sagittal anorectoplasty. J Pediatr Surg 1982;5: 638–43.
6. Georgeson KE, Inge TH, Albanese CT. Laparoscopically assisted anorectal pull-through for high imperforate anus—a new technique. J Pediatr Surg 2000;35(6): 927–31.
7. Cuschieri A. Descriptive epidemiology of isolated anal anomalies: a survey of 4.6 million births in Europe. Am J Med Genet 2001;103:207–15.
8. Schramm C, Draaken M, Tewes G, et al. Autosomal-dominant non-syndromic anal atresia: sequencing of candidate genes, array-based molecular karyotyping, and review of the literature. Eur J Pediatr 2011;170(6):741–6.
9. Rooij IA, Wijers CH, Rieu PN, et al. Maternal and paternal risk factors for anorectal malformations: a Dutch case-control study. Birth Defects Res A Clin Mol Teratol 2010;88(3):152–8.
10. Sadler TW. Langman's medical embryology. 8th edition: Lippincott, Williams & Wilkins; 2000. p. 297–301.
11. Holschneider AM, Hutson JM. Anorectal malformations in children. Berlin: Springer; 2006. p. 49–55.
12. Marcelis C, de Blaauw I, Brunner H. Chromosomal anomalies in the etiology of anorectal malformations: a review. Am J Med Genet Part A 2011;155:2692–704.
13. Mundt E, Bates MD. Genetics of Hirschsprung disease and anorectal malformations. Semin Pediatr Surg 2010;19:107–17.
14. Suda H, Lee KJ, Semba K, et al. The Skt gene, required for anorectal development is a candidate for a molecular marker of the cloacal plate. Pediatr Surg Int 2011;27:269–73.
15. Zhang J, Zhang ZB, Gao H, et al. Down regulation of SHH/BMP4 signaling in human anorectal malformations. J Int Med Res 2009;37:1842–50.
16. Tai CC, Sala FG, Ford HR, et al. Wnt5a knock-out mouse as a new model of anorectal malformation. J Surg Res 2009;156:278–82.
17. Bekhit E, Murphy F, Puri P, et al. The clinical features and diagnostic guideline for identification of anorectal malformations. In: Holschneider AM, Hutson JM,

editors. Anorectal malformations in children. Berlin: Springer; 2006. p. 185. Chapter 9.

18. Wangensteen OH, Rice CO. Imperforate anus: a method of determining the surgical approach. Ann Surg 1930;92:77–81.
19. Narasimharao KL, Prasad GR, Katariya S, et al. Prone cross table lateral view: an alternative to the invertogrqam in imperforate anus. AJR Am J Roentgenol 1983; 140:227–9.
20. Stoll C, Alembik Y, Dott B, et al. Associated malformations in patients with anorectal anomalies. Eur J Med Genet 2007;50:281–90.
21. Teixeira OH, Malhotra K, Sellers J, et al. Cardiovascular anomalies with imperforate anus. Arch Dis Child 1983;58:747–9.
22. Orun UA, Bilci M, Demirceken FG, et al. Gastrointestinal system malformation in children area associated with congenital heart defects. Anadolu Kardiyol Derg 2011;11(2):146–9.
23. Suppiej A, Dal Zotto L, Cappellari A, et al. Tethered cord in patients with anorectal malformation; preliminary results. Pediatr Surg Int 2009;10:851–5.
24. Golonka NR, Hag LJ, Keating RP, et al. Routine MRI evaluation of low imperforate anus reveals unexpected high incidence of tethered spinal cord. J Pediatr Surg 2002;37:966–9.
25. Nievelstein RA, Vos A, Valk J, et al. Magnetic resonance imaging in children with anorectal malformations: embryologic implications. J Pediatr Surg 2002;37(8): 1138–45.
26. Ratan SK, Rattn KN, Pandey RM, et al. Associated congenital anomalies in patients with anorectal malformations-a need for developing a uniform practical approach. J Pediatr Surg 2004;39(11):1706–11.
27. Warne SA, Godley ML, Owens CM, et al. The validity of sacral ratios to identify sacral abnormalities. BJU Int 2003;91(6):540–4.
28. Currarino G, Coln D, Votteler T. Triad of anorectal, sacral, and presacral anomalies. Am J Roentgenol 1981;137(2):395–8.
29. Inomata Y, Tanaka K, Ozawa K. Sacral anomaly and pelvic floor muscle in imperforate anus: a clinical and experimental study. Nihon Geka Hokan 1989;58(2): 217–30.
30. Rintala RJ, Lindahl H. Is normal bowel function possible after repair of intermediate and high anorectal malformations? J Pediatr Surg 1995;30:491–4.
31. Peña A. Anorectal malformations. Semin Pediatr Surg 1995;4(1):35–47.
32. McLorie BA, Sheldon CA, Fleisher M, et al. The genitourinary system in patients with imperforate anus. J Pediatr Surg 1987;22(12):1100–4.
33. Goossens WJ, Blaauw I, Wijnen MH, et al. Urological anomalies in anorectal malformations in the Netherlands: effect of screening all patients on long term outcome. Pediatr Surg Int 2011;27:1091–7.
34. Boemers TM, Bax KM, Rovekamp MH, et al. The effect of posterior sagittal anorectoplasty and its variants on lower urinary tract function in children with anorectal malformations. J Urol 1995;153:191–3.
35. Senel E, Akbiyik F, Atayurt H. Urological problems or fecal continence during long term follow up of patients with anorectal malformation. Pediatr Surg Int 2010;26: 683–9.
36. Levitt MA, Bischoff A, Breech L, et al. Rectovestibular fistula-rarely recognized associated gynecologic anomalies. J Pediatr Surg 2009;44:1261–7.
37. Coran AG, Graziano K. Vaginal reconstruction for congenital and acquired abnormalities. In: Holschneider AM, Hutson JM, editors. Anorectal malformations in children. Berlin (Heidelberg): Springer; 2006. p. 445. Chapter 35.

38. Levitt MA, Stein DM, Peña A. Rectovestibular fistula with absent vagina: a unique anorectal malformation. J Pediatr Surg 1998;33(7):986–90.
39. Minto CL, Hollings N, Hall Cragggs M, et al. Magnetic resonance imaging in the assessment of complex müllerian anomalies. BJOG 2001;108:791–7.
40. Murphy F, Puri P, Hutson J, et al. Incidence and frequency of different types and classification of anorectal malformations. In: Holschneider AM, Hutson JM, editors. Anorectal malformations in children. Berlin (Heidelberg): Springer; 2006. p. 173.
41. Gross GW, Wolfson PJ, Peña A. Augmented-pressure colostogram in imperforate anus with fistula. Pediatr Radiol 1991;21:560–2.
42. Hong AR, Acuna MF, Peña A, et al. Urologic injuries associated with repair of anorectal malformation in male patients. J Pediatr Surg 2002;3:339–44.
43. Levitt A, Peña M. Imperforate anus and cloacal malformations. In: Holcomb GW, Murphy JP. Ashcraft's pediatric surgery. 5th edition. Philadelphia (PA): Saunders Elsevier; 2010. p. 469. Chapter 36.
44. Bischoff A, Levitt MA, Peña A. Laparoscopy and its use in the repair of anorectal malformations. J Pediatr Surg 2011;46:1609–17.
45. Bailez MM, Cuenca ES, DiBenedetto V, et al. Laparoscopic treatment of rectovaginal fistulas. feasibility, technical details and functional results of a rare anorectal malformation. J Pediatr Surg 2010;45:1837–42.
46. Bailez MM, Cuenca ES, Mauri V, et al. Outcome of males with high anorectal malformations treated with laparoscopic-assisted anorectal pull-through preliminary results of a comparative study with the open approach in single institution. J Pediatr Surg 2011;46:473–7.
47. Peña A, Grasshoff S, Levitt M. Reoperations in anorectal malformations. J Pediatr Surg 2007;42:318–25.
48. Potts WJ. Imperforate anus and associated anomalies. Pediatr Clin North Am 1956;67–77.
49. Peña A. Total urogenital mobilization—an easier way to repair cloacas. J Pediatr Surg 1997;32:263–8.
50. Belizon A, Levitt MA, Shoshany G, et al. Rectal prolapse following posterior sagittal anorectoplasty for anorectal malformations. J Pediatr Surg 2005;40:192–6.
51. Rintala RJ, Pakarinen MP. Outcome of anorectal malformations and Hirschsprung's disease beyond childhood. Semin Pediatr Surg 2010;19:160–7.
52. Hashish MS, Dawoud HH, Hirschl RB, et al. Long-term functional outcome and quality of life in patients with high imperforate anus. J Pediatr Surg 2010;45(1):224–30.
53. Levitt MA, Kant A, Peña A. The morbidity of constipation in patients with anorectal malformations. J Pediatr Surg 2010;45:1228–33.
54. Rintala RJ, Lindahl HG. Fecal continence in patient having undergone posterior sagittal anorectoplasty procedure for a high anorectal malformation improves at adolescence, as constipation disappears. J Pediatr Surg 2001;36:1218–21.

Index

Note: Page numbers of article titles are in **boldface** type.

Clin Perinatol 39 (2012) 423–430
doi:10.1016/S0095-5108(12)00038-3
0095-5108/12/$ – see front matter © 2012 Elsevier Inc. All rights reserved.

perinatology.theclinics.com

Moving?

Make sure your subscription moves with you!

To notify us of your new address, find your **Clinics Account Number** (located on your mailing label above your name), and contact customer service at:

Email: journalscustomerservice-usa@elsevier.com

800-654-2452 (subscribers in the U.S. & Canada)
314-447-8871 (subscribers outside of the U.S. & Canada)

Fax number: 314-447-8029

Elsevier Health Sciences Division
Subscription Customer Service
3251 Riverport Lane
Maryland Heights, MO 63043

*To ensure uninterrupted delivery of your subscription, please notify us at least 4 weeks in advance of move.

Printed and bound by CPI Group (UK) Ltd, Croydon, CR0 4YY

03/10/2024

01040457-0018